17.99

A guide for health & beauty therapists
Volume 2
The body

Gaynor Winyard

An imprint of Pearson Education

Harlow, England · London · New York · Reading, Massachusetts · San Francisco
Toronto · Don Mills, Ontario · Sydney · Tokyo · Singapore · Hong Kong · Seoul
Taipei · Cape Town · Madrid · Mexico City · Amsterdam · Munich · Paris · Milan

Pearson Education Limited
Edinburgh Gate
Harlow
Essex CM20 2JE
England

and Associated Companies throughout the world

Visit us on the World Wide Web at :
http://www.pearsoneduc.com

First published 1992

10   9   8   7
05   04   03   02   01

ISBN 0 582 413613

British Library Cataloguing in Publication Data
A catalogue record for this book is available from the
British Library.

Set by 3 in Linotron Times Roman 9/10

Printed in Malaysia (PP)

Contents

Acknowledgements

We are grateful to the following for permission to reproduce copyright material:

Churchill Livingstone for the following figures from *Anatomy and physiology in health and illness* by J. S. Ross and K. J. W. Wilson: our figures, 1.2 (a), 1.2 (b), 1.4, 1.5, 1.6, 1.7 (b), 1.8, 1.9, 1.10, 1.11, 1.14 (a), 1.14 (b), 1.15, 1.16, 3.1, 3.2 (a), 3.2 (b), 3.3, 3.4, 3.5, 3.6, 3.7, 3.8, 3.9, 3.10, 3.11, 3.12, 3.13, 3.14, 3.15, 3.16, 3.17, 3.18, 3.19, 3.20, 3.21, 3.22, 3.23, 3.24, 3.25, 3.26, 3.27, 4.1, 4.2, 4.3, 4.4, 4.5, 4.6, 4.7, 4.8, 4.9, 4.10, 4.11, 4.12, 4.13, 4.14, 5.1, 5.2, 5.3, 5.4, 5.5, 5.6, 5.7, 5.8, 5.9, 5.10, 6.1, 6.2, 6.3, 6.4, 6.5, 6.6, 6.7, 6.8, 6.9, 6.10, 6.11, 6.12, 6.13, 7.1, 7.2, 7.3, 7.4, 7.5, 7.6, 7.7, 7.8, 7.9, 13.4 (a), 13.4 (b), Health and Beauty Equipment Centre, Holloway, London for our Fig. 11.5.

Thanks are also due to Mike Devlin, who took the photographs, and Grace Andrews, for her help and encouragement.

Chapter 1

Support and movement

The skeletal system of the body consists of the *bones* which support the body, the *articulations* or joints between those bones, and the skeletal *muscles* which are attached to the bones. Contraction of the muscles causes movement of the bones at the joints. The bony skeleton and the muscles also combine to protect the organs in the *main cavities of the body*.

Bones

The bony skeleton may be considered in two parts, *The axial skeleton* with 80 bones forming the upright axis of the body, and *the appendicular skeleton* which consists of the 64 bones of the upper extremity and the 62 bones of the lower extremity. The term 'extremity' includes both the limbs and the girdles by which the limbs are attached to the axial skeleton.

The axial skeleton (see Table 1.1)

This consists of the skull, spinal column, sternum and ribs.

The bones of the skull

There are 8 in the cranium and 14 in the face and these have been detailed in Vol. 1 (Chap. 4). Associated with this area are three bones in each ear (malleus, incus and stapes) and the hyoid bone in the throat, though these small bones rarely concern the beauty therapist.

The spinal column

This is a flexible structure comprising a number of bones called vertebrae. There are 26 vertebral bones (or 33 before fusion of bones to form the sacrum and coccyx) and these are segmented according to the region they occupy. There are:

- 7 cervical vertebrae, which form the skeletal framework of the neck and cervical area;
- 12 thoracic vertebrae in the posterior part of the chest to which 12 pairs of ribs are attached;

Table 1.1 Summary of axial skeleton (80 bones)

Location	No. of bones	Name			
Skull	22	Cranium	8 i.e.	Frontal	1
				Parietal	1
				Temporal	2
				Occipital	1
				Sphenoid	1
				Ethmoid	1
		Facial	14	Nasal	2
				Maxillary	2
				Zygomatic	2
				Mandible	1
				Lacrimal	2
				Palatine	2
				Turbinate	2
				Vomer	1
Ears	6			Malleus	2
				Incus	2
				Stapes	2
Throat	1	Hyoid			
Spinal column	26	Vertebrae	24	Cervical	7
				Thoracic	12
				Lumbar	5
		Sacrum	1		
		Coccyx	1		
Chest	1	Sternum			
Ribs	24	True ribs	(Pairs)	7	
		False	(Pairs)	5 of which 2 pairs are floating ribs	

- 5 lumbar vertebrae that support the small of the back;
- 1 sacrum which is a wedge-shaped bone in an adult of approximately 25 years or more, but before fusion was originally 5 separate vertebrae;
- 1 coccyx, a single bone, but again 4 separate vertebrae in childhood (see Fig. 1.1).

The vertebrae in the three upper regions remain distinct and generally separate throughout life and are called moveable vertebrae. The sacrum and coccyx are termed fixed vertebrae.

Generally most vertebrae resemble each other but there are differences. The anterior part of the vertebrae (with the exception of the first two cervical vertebrae) consists of a body which is a flat, round mass, cylindrical in structure and which is the weight-bearing part of the vertebrae. These bodies are separated above and below by discs of cartilage and fibrous tissue. These intervertebral discs act as cushions to absorb mechanical shocks, i.e. running, jogging etc. Rupture of an intervertebral disc is commonly known as a 'slipped disc' and may, in extreme cases, need surgery.

The posterior part of a vertebra consists of two short, thick processes projecting backwards from the body and these are called *pedicles*. Projecting from the ends of the pedicles are two bony plates known as *laminae*. These join together to form a semi-circular arch – the *neural* arch, which encloses a foramen (a natural opening) known as a vertebral or spinal foramen. (Spina bifida is the result of an imperfect union or congenital absence of one or more neural arches.)

Vertebral foramina of all the vertebrae are aligned to form a spinal cavity to house the spinal cord. From the union of the laminae and pedicles there are right and left lateral projections known as *transverse processes* and these give attachment to muscles and ligaments. Posteriorly, where the two laminae unite, there is a large, backward-pointing projection of bone, called the *spinous process*. This can be felt down the middle of the back and also gives attachment to muscles and ligaments. There are also articulating processes, i.e. superior (which project upward from the laminae), and inferior (which project downward from the laminae and therefore articulate with the superior articulating processes of the vertebrae below and limit rotation of the vertebral column).

The cervical vertebrae   The first and second cervical have been described in Vol. 1 (Chap. 4) but to summarise:

- The atlas (1st vertebra) lacks body and spinous process. It forms a hinge joint with the condyles of the occipital bone of the skull which allows nodding movements of the head.
- The axis (2nd vertebra) forms a pivot for the atlas to allow rotation of the head.
- The bodies of the other cervical vertebrae are small and oblong, broad from side to side and the spinal foramina are large and triangular. The exception is the seventh cervical vertebra where the spinous process is longer and this can be felt when the head is bent forward.

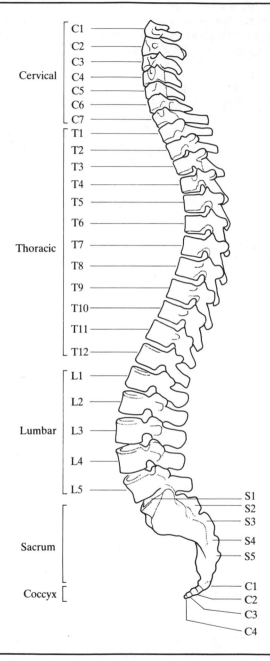

Fig. 1.1 Bones of the vertebrae

The thoracic vertebrae These 12 thoracic vertebrae have a typical structure but with special facets at each side which articulate with the twelve pairs of ribs. For a typical vertebra see Fig. 1.2(a) and Fig. 1.2(b).

The lumbar vertebrae These five lumbar vertebrae are strong, as they bear the weight of the upper body. The spinous processes are short. The superior articulating processes are directed inwards instead of upwards and the inferior articulating processes are directed outward instead of downward (see Fig. 1.3(a) and Fig. 1.3(b)).

The sacrum The sacrum is a triangular bone which consists of five vertebrae fused together to form a flattened plate of bone (see Fig. 1.4). It is wedged dorsally between the two innominate bones (see pelvic girdle) and forms the

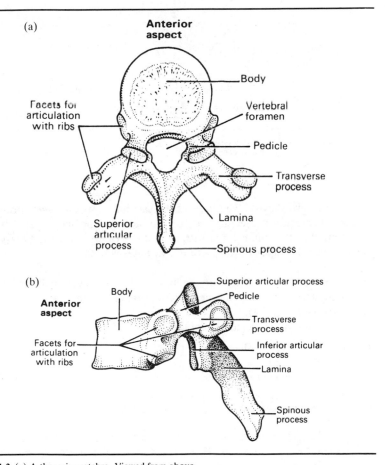

Fig. 1.2 (a) A thoracic vertebra. Viewed from above
(b) A thoracic vertebra. Viewed from the side

(a)

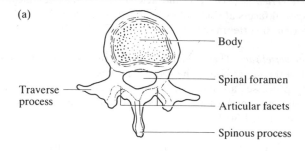

Body

Spinal foramen

Traverse process

Articular facets

Spinous process

(b)

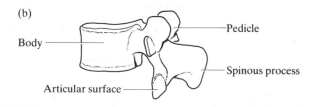

Pedicle

Body

Spinous process

Articular surface

Fig. 1.3 (a) Lumbar vertebra: upper aspect
(b) Lumbar vertebra: lateral aspect

back of the pelvic cavity. The base of the sacrum forms the sacral promontory, i.e. the upper projecting part of the sacrum. The sacral canal is the continuation of the spinal canal with its walls perforated for the passage of sacral nerves. The apex of the sacrum articulates with the coccyx.

The coccyx The coccyx lies at the base of the vertebral column and is composed of four or five vertebrae fused to form one bone. It articulates with the sacrum (see Fig. 1.4).

The functions of the vertebral column are to:

- contain and protect the spinal cord;
- support the head;
- support and permit movement of the trunk;
- give attachments to the upper and lower limbs, ribs and muscles;
- act as a shock absorber.

Curves of the vertebral column To make the balance possible in the upright position and to carry the strength of the vertebral column, the spinal column is curved. There are four curves and these are named according to their location. From the side view, the cervical curve is convex anteriorly; the

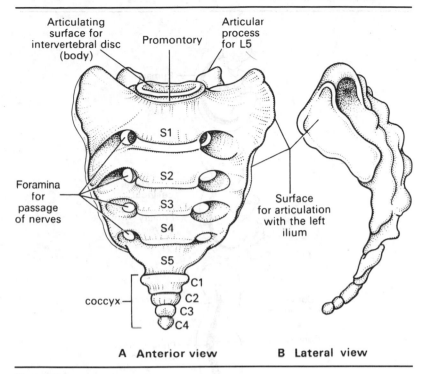

Fig. 1.4 The sacrum and coccyx

thoracic curve is concave anteriorly; the lumbar curve is convex anteriorly; and the sacral curve is concave anteriorly (see Fig. 1.5).

At birth, a baby has a continuous posterior convexity, i.e. a 'C'-shaped rounded back from head to coccyx. This is called the primary curve and the thoracic and sacral spine retain this curve throughout life. As the infant grows the neck curves forward and the head can be raised. This is the first of the secondary curves. As the child begins to walk, secondary curves develop in the lumbar region.

It is not uncommon the for spinal curves to deviate from the normal. For example:

- kyphosis is an abnormally increased *posterior* convexity in the curvature of the thoracic spine resembling a 'hunchback';
- *lordosis* is the abnormally increased *posterior* concavity in the curvature of the lumbar spine;
- scoliosis is a lateral curvature of the spine. In Chapter 2 (pp. 44) when posture is observed this condition may be recognized as it is often a cause of habitually poor posture over a long period of time. It can also be accompanied by a lack of muscle tone and physical inactivity.

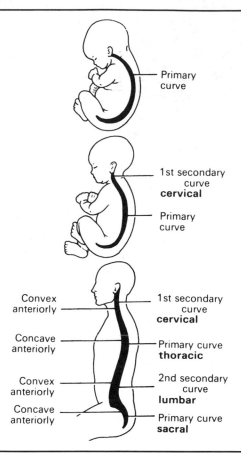

Fig. 1.5 Diagram showing the order of development of the curves of the spine

The sternum

The medial part of the anterior chest wall is supported by the sternum or breast-bone. It articulates with the clavicles and the cartilages of the first seven ribs and is divided into three parts:

- The manubrium sterni, which is a triangular-shaped bone placed above the body of the sternum. The first pair of ribs articulate with the sides of the manubrium. The second pair of ribs articulate at the junction of the manubrium and the body of the sternum. This junction is called the *angle of Louis* or *the angle of Ludwig.*
- The body of the sternum is long and narrow. It is notched on either side forming facets for the attachment of costal cartilages of the 3rd, 4th, 5th, 6th and 7th ribs.
- The *Xiphoid* process is a cartilaginous plate which is the lowest part of

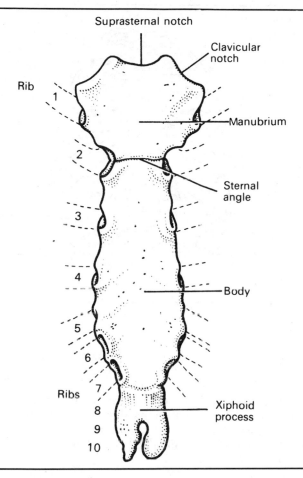

Fig. 1.6 The sternum and its attachments

the sternum. The diaphragm and rectus abdominis muscles and linea alba (explained later) are attached to the Xiphoid process.

The ribs

The vertebral column, sternum and 12 pairs of ribs form the bony cage known as the *thorax* (see Fig. 1.7(a)). Each rib is a long 'C'-shaped bone which has two extremities, anterior and posterior, and a shaft. The posterior extremity which attaches itself to the vertebra has a head, a neck and a tubercle (i.e. small eminence). The anterior or sternal end has a depression for the attachment of the costal cartilage. The rib articulates posteriorly with both the body and the transverse process of its corresponding thoracic vertebra (see Fig. 1.7(b)). From the vertebrae the ribs slope forward and

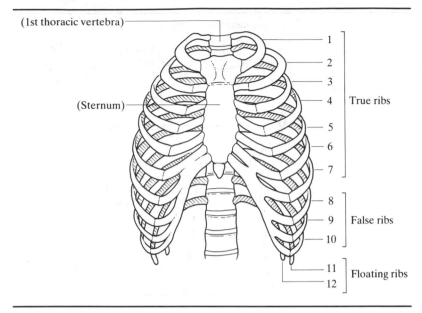

(1st thoracic vertebra)

(Sternum)

1
2
3
4 True ribs
5
6
7

8
9 False ribs
10

11 Floating ribs
12

Fig. 1.7 (a) Thorax (anterior aspect)

downward. The upper seven pairs of ribs are attached to the sternum anteriorly by means of their costal cartilages and are termed the *true ribs*. Each of the costal cartilages of the next three ribs (8th, 9th and 10th) fuse with the cartilage of the rib above and are termed *false ribs*. The 11th and 12th ribs are termed *floating ribs* as they are not, even indirectly, attached to the sternum.

The costal cartilages are ridges of hyaline cartilage connecting the ribs to the sternum and serve to protect the sternum from injury.

The function of the rib cage is to:

- give shape to the thorax;
- protect the principal organs in the thoracic cavity and upper abdomen;
- support the upper limbs through the sternum;
- alter the volume of the thorax causing breathing;
- give attachment to many muscles.

The appendicular skeleton (see Table 1.2)

The upper extremity consists of the bones of the shoulder girdle (clavicle and scapula), upper arm (humerus), lower arm (radius and ulna), wrist (carpals) and hand (metacarpals and phalanges). All have been described in Vol. 1 (Chaps 4 and 18).

The lower extremity consists of the pelvic girdle and the bone of the thigh (femur), the lower leg (tibia and fibula), and knee cap (patella), the ankle

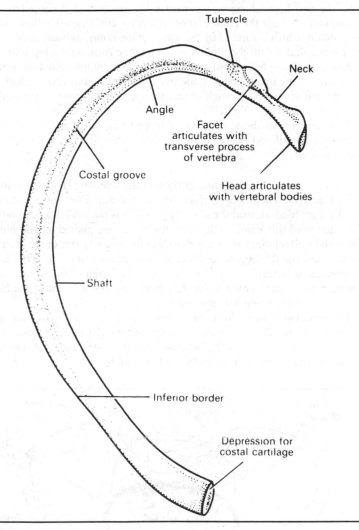

Fig. 1.7 (b) A typical rib viewed from below

bones (tarsals) and the bones of the foot (metatarsals and phalanges). The bones of the lower leg, ankle and foot have been described in Vol. 1 (Chap. 23).

The pelvic girdle

This is a stable circular base which supports the trunk and the lower limbs and it is formed by the two innominate bones and part of the axial skeleton (i.e. the sacrum and coccyx). Each innominate bone is large and irregularly shaped and articulates in front with the corresponding bone of the opposite side, the two bones forming a considerable part of the bony pelvis. On its lateral surface, near the middle, there is a deep, cup-shaped hollow called the acetabulum which is formed by the union of the ilium, ischium and the pubis. It also articulates with the thigh bone (femur) so forming the hip joint. There is a large oval gap below and in front of the acetabulum called the obturator foramen. Strong ligaments bind the two innominate bones, posteriorly to the sacrum and anteriorly to each other; the sacrum and coccyx are wedged in between dorsally (see Fig. 1.8).

Each innominate bone consists of three parts which are separated by a cartilage in childhood but are united by bone in an adult (see Fig. 1.9). These are as follows.

The ilium   is the lateral, flaring portion of the hip bone. It has two surfaces, a crest and an articulating surface for the sacrum. The upper extremity is greatly expanded to form the iliac crest, which is the curved upper border of the ilium, and this can be felt when the hands are placed on the hips. The ilium gives attachment to many muscles and includes the upper part of the acetabulum and the expanded, flattened area of bone above it. The iliac crest terminates anteriorly at one of the four iliac spines, called the anterior superior iliac spine, which can be felt externally as the point of the hip, and posteriorly in the posterior superior iliac spine.

The other two spines, the anterior and posterior inferior spines are situated just below these. The articulating surface for the sacrum lies between the two posterior spines and below this articulation is the sciatic notch, through which the sciatic nerve passes through to the lower limbs.

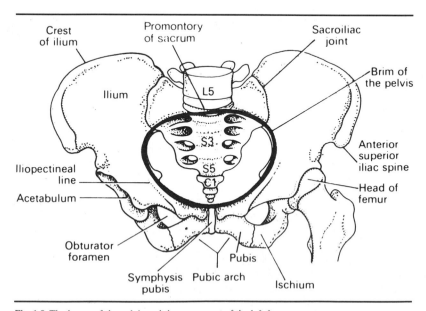

Fig. 1.8 The bones of the pelvis and the upper part of the left femur

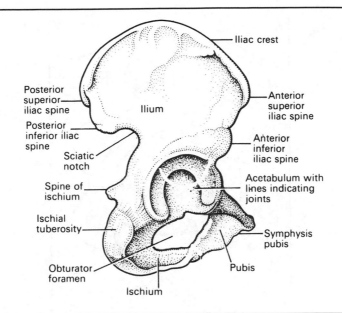

Fig. 1.9 The right innominate bone. Lateral view

The pubis forms the ventral part of the innominate bone and meets the opposite pubis in front to form a cartilaginous joint, called the pubic symphysis. The pubis has a body which is square with a free upper border termed the pubic crest and two rami, i.e. the inferior ramus which fuses with the ramus of ischium and the superior ramus which extends from the body to the acetabulum.

The ischium is the lower, posterior part of the innominate bone. It has a body and a ramus. The upper extremity of the body forms the lower and posterior part of the acetabulum. The ramus of ischium projects from the lower extremity and fuses with the inferior ramus of pubis to complete the obturator foramen. The ischial tuberosity is the large, rough, quadrilateral process on which the trunk rests when the body is erect in a sitting position. Just above this tuberosity is a pointed prominence at the back of the bone termed the ischial spine and this marks the lowest part of the sciatic notch.

Pelvic structure in men and women differ in size and shape. The female hips are wider and the pelvic cavity is round, relatively large and constructed to accommodate the foetus during pregnancy. The male pelvic cavity is heart-shaped, narrow and proportionately heavier and stronger (see Fig. 1.10).

The femur (see Fig. 1.11)
This is the longest and strongest bone in the body and is situated in the thigh.

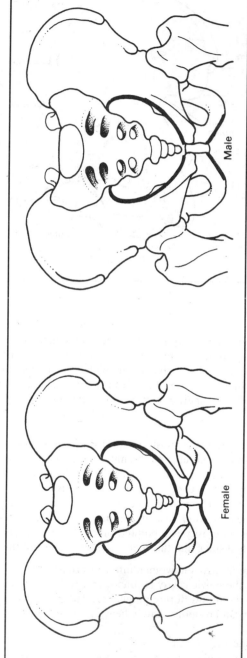

Fig. 1.10 Diagram showing the difference in shape of the male and female pelvis

It articulates proximally with the acetabulum and distally with the patella and tibia. It is a long bone with a shaft and two extremities.

The shaft is cylindrical and smooth. It is rounded at the front and sides and its posterior border has a marked ridge, called the linea aspera, to which numerous muscles are attached.

The upper extremity of the femur comprises:

● a head, which is rounded (i.e. forming rather more than half a 'sphere') and is directed upwards, medially and slightly forwards to articulate with the acetabulum;

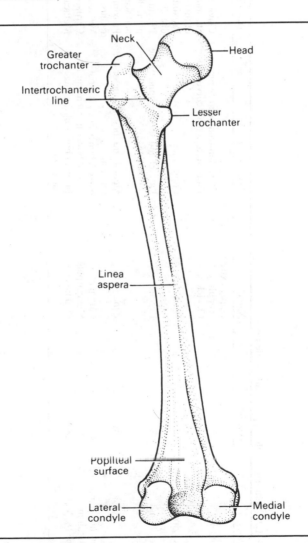

Fig. 1.11 The left femur. Posterior aspect

Table 1.2 Summary of the appendicular skeleton

Location	No. bones	Name	Description	Articulates with:
		Upper extremity (64 bones)		
Shoulder	2	Scapula	Wide thin triangular bone	Clavicle and humerus
	2	Clavicle	Elongated slender curved bone	Sternum, scapula and cartilage of first rib
Upper arms	2	Humerus	Long bone	Proximally with scapula, distally with radius and ulna
Lower arms	2	Radius	Lateral and shorter bone of the forearm	Proximally with humerus and ulna, distally with ulna, lunate and scaphoid bones
	2	Ulna	Medial and longer bone of the forearm	Proximally with humerus and radius, distally with radius
Wrists and hands (In detail in Chap. 18, Vol. 1)	16	Carpals	8 small bones in each wrist	Metacarpals and radius
	10	Metacarpals	5 small bones in each hand	Carpals and phalanges
	28	Phalanges	14 small bones of the fingers in each hand	Metacarpals

Lower extremity (62 bones)

Hips and pelvis 2	Innominate (3 parts) Ilium		Broad lateral part of innominate bone	
	Ischium		Lower thick three-sided posterior part of innominate bone	Union of three bones at the acetabulum which receives the head of the femur
	Pubis		Ventral part of innominate bone	
Thighs	Femur	2	Long bone of the thigh	Proximally with the acetabulum, distally with patella and tibia
Knees	Patella	2	Small sesamoid bone over anterior aspect of the knee	Femur
Lower leg	Tibia	2	Medial and larger bone of the lower leg	Proximally with femur and fibula, distally with talus and fibula
(In detail in Chap. 23 Vol. 1)	Fibula	2	Lateral and smaller bone of the lower leg	Proximally with tibia, distally with tibia and talus
	Tarsals	14	7 small bones in the ankle and foot	Tibia, fibula and metatarsals
	Metatarsals	10	5 small bones in each foot	Tarsals and phalanges
	Phalanges	28	14 small bones in the toes of each foot	Metatarsals

- a neck, which is the constricted part just below the head, and which connects the head and shaft and forms an angle of about 125°; this allows the lower limb considerable movement;
- the greater trochanter, which is a large protuberance located inferiorly and laterally at the upper part of the junction of the neck with the shaft;
- the lesser trochanter, which is a small protuberance located inferiorly and medially with the lower and posterior part of the neck.

The lower extremity of the femur comprises two condyles, which are large, rounded masses of bone, one on the medial and one on the lateral surface of the femur and both enter into the formation of the knee joint. Anteriorly, the two condyles are united but posteriorly they are separated by the intercondylar notch. Cruciate (or cross-shaped) ligaments that help to bind the femur to the tibia are found in this notch. The patella itself rests on the patella surface which extends over the anterior aspect of both condyles and the popliteal surface of the bone lies above the condyles posteriorly and forms the floor of the popliteal space.

The names and number of bones in the appendicular skeleton are summarised in Table 1.2.

Articulation

An articulation is the place of union or junction between two or more bones and the primary function of a joint is to provide motion and flexibility for the skeleton.

The classification of joints

This has been briefly described in Vol. 1 (Chap. 3). To expand further:

1. fibrous joints (also known as synarthroses) are immovable or fixed joints, e.g. where segments of bone are fused together as in the skull;
2. cartilaginous joints (also known as amphiarthroses) allow limited movement and these include the following:

- The joints of the vertebral column where there is only slight movement between adjacent lower cervical, thoracic and lumbar vertebrae. The intervertebral discs are thickest in the lumbar region and thinner in the thoracic region. However, the total amount of slight movement over the length of the vertebral column allows considerable flexibility.
- The joint between the manubrium and the body of the sternum.
- The pubic symphysis where cartilage unites the two pubic bones. As a matter of interest, during childbirth, slight movement at the symphysis pubis facilitates the baby's passage through the pelvis.
- There are also primary cartilaginous joints found between the diaphysis and epiphyses of the long bones in childhood.

3. synovial joints (also known as diathroses) are freely movable joints. The

six varieties have been described in Vol. 1 (Chap. 3) and Table 1.3 gives a summary of the main synovial joints.

If any of these synovial joints are examined it will be seen that the surfaces are covered with hyaline cartilage which fit together accurately. There is an exception, the genual or knee joint. The condyles of the femur are round and the upper extremity of the tibia is flat. Very small half-moon wedges of cartilage lie between the two surfaces, shaping the upper end of the tibia and rounding the surface to fit the condyles of the femur. These cartilages may be torn as a result of injury to the knee, a condition commonly found in footballers and miners.

In all synovial joints the bones are held together by a cuff of fibrous tissue. This is called the capsule and, in certain situations, it is strengthened by ligaments. A sprain is the condition resulting from the tearing of some of the fibres of a ligament. A more serious condition results when the whole ligament is torn, as this may produce a dislocation which is the displacement of the joint surface.

The joint capsule has a smooth lining of synovial membrane. This membrane secretes the fluid which keeps the joints lubricated. It also covers all surfaces inside the joint capsule which are not already covered with hyaline cartilage. This provides movement without friction. These joints are meant to be moved and fixation, for any reason, will result in stiffness and pain. *Ankylosis* is immobility and solidification of a joint.

Joints are also subject to inflammation, the most prevalent types are *osteoarthritis*, a degenerative joint disorder common to elderly people and *rheumatoid arthritis* which may even occur in the very young.

As a beauty therapist there is very little you can do, except temporarily relieve the pain with the application of paraffin wax or, better still, parafango wax (described in Chapter 14).

Movements in joints

These can be gliding, angular, rotary and circumductory.

Gliding movements
These are formed by the opposition of plane surfaces and the movement has no definite axis, e.g. between the tarsal bones in the feet, and the carpal bones at the wrist.

Angular movements
Angular movements produce an increase of the angle between two bones. Two antagonistic or opposite movements are often possible, e.g. flexion and extension, eversion and inversion, abduction and adduction, and elevation and depression.

Flexion means a decrease of the angle or bending, e.g. flexion of the vertebrae causes forward bending of the trunk. Lateral flexion of the vertebrae

Table 1.3 Summary of synovial joints

	Joints	Articulation	Movement
1. Gliding	Sterno-clavicular	Medial end of the clavicle with the clavicular notch of the manubrium sterni	Gliding
	Acromio-clavicular	Distal end of the clavicle with the acromion process of the scapula	Slight gliding movements possible between clavicle and scapula
	Carpo-metacarpal	Distal aspect of the lower row of carpal bones with the five metacarpal bones	Gliding
	Tibio-fibular	Head of the fibula with the lateral condyle of the tibia	Gliding
	Talo-calcaneal	Between talus and calcaneum	Slight rocking
	Medio-tarsal	Between head of talus and navicular and between calcaneum and cuboid	Inversion and eversion
2. Ball and socket	Humero-scapular	Head of humerus (forming one-third of sphere) within the glenoid cavity. Latter is deepened by attachment of a fibro-cartilage rim – the glenoid labrum. Bones are united by ligaments so forming a loose capsule.	Dependent on surrounding muscles, abduction, adduction flexion, extension, medial and lateral rotation (Circumduction)
	Coxal (hip)	Head of femur in acetabulum of the innominate bone. Acetabulum is deepened by attachment of the acetabular labrum fibro-cartilage	Flexion, extension, abduction adduction, medial and lateral rotation (Circumduction)
3. Condyle	Radio-carpal	Lower end of the radius and articular disc below the head of the ulna and scaphoid, lunate and triquetral bones	Flexion, extension, abduction, and adduction of hand

Type	Joint	Articulation	Movement
3. Condyle (cont'd)	Metacarpal-phalangeal	Distal end of the metacarpals with the proximal end of the phalanges	Flexion, extension, abduction, adduction of hand
	Interphalangeal	Heads of the proximal phalanges into articulating surfaces on the bases of the distal phalanges	Flexion, extension
	Tarso-metatarsal	Distal end of the metatarsals with the proximal end of the phalanges	Flexion, extension, abduction, adduction of foot
	Interphalangeal	Heads of the proximal phalanges into articulating surfaces on the bases of the distal phalanges	Flexion, extension
4. Hinge	Humero-ulna	Trochlear surface on lower extremity of humerus and trochlear notch of ulna	Flexion and extension
	Cubital (elbow) Humero-radial	Head of radius with the capitulum of humerus	Flexion and extension
	Genual (knee)	Distal end of the femur and proximal end of the tibia	Flexion, extension, slight medial rotation
5. Pivot	Atlanto-axial	Anterior arch of atlas rotates about the dens of the axis	Pivots
	Cubital (elbow) radio-ulnar	Head of radius in radial notch	Supination and pronation of lower arm and hand in rotation
6. Saddle	Carpo-metacarpal	Proximal end of first metacarpal and trapezium	Moves in several directions

(side flexion) involves movement of the vertebral column when any part of it bends sideways, either at the waist (lumbar), neck (cervical), or in the middle of the back (thoracic). Flexion of the ankle brings the dorsum of the foot up towards the leg (dorsi-flexion).

Extension   involves increasing the angle or straightening. Extension of the vertebrae causes straightening of the spine. Extension of the ankle stretches the foot down from the ankle joint (also known as plantar flexion due to the raising of the heel).

Eversion   means turning outwards (laterally), e.g. when the sole of the foot is turned to face outwards.

Inversion   means turning inwards (medially), e.g. when the sole of the foot is turned to face inwards.

Abduction   means moving away from the mid-line, e.g. when limbs move away from the mid-line of the body or when fingers move away from the mid-line of the hand.

Adduction   is a movement towards the mid-line of the body or of the fingers towards the mid-line of the hand.

Elevation   is an upward movement, e.g. when the shoulder girdle is raised. When the arm is abducted to shoulder level, the movement which takes the arm from this point up towards the side of the head and ear is *abduction through elevation*. When the arm is flexed to shoulder level, the movement which takes the arm upwards to the side of the head and ear is *elevation through flexion*.

Depression   is a movement downwards, e.g. at the temporomandibular joint when the mouth is opened.

Rotary movements

Rotation   is when a bone moves around its long axis, or when one bone pivots around another, e.g. as in the medial and lateral rotation of the upper bone of the arm (humerus) or when the atlas vertebra rotates on the pivot formed by the dens of the axis vertebra.

Pronation   is the act of assuming the prone position, i.e. lying face downwards. It also applies to the hand by rotating the radius on the ulna until the hand lies palm downwards.

Supination   is the act of assuming a supine position, i.e. lying face upwards. It also applies to the hand by the act of turning the palm upwards.

Circumductory movements

Circumduction is a combination of the angular movements. The hip and shoulder joints are examples of this kind of movement, in which large circles of movement can be performed.

Muscles

Muscle tissue and various muscles have been detailed in Vol. 1. For easy reference, see

face muscles	Vol. 1, Table 4.1
neck and shoulder girdle muscles	Vol. 1, Table 4.2
arm muscles	Vol. 1, Table 18.1
hand muscles	Vol. 1, Table 18.2
lower leg muscles	Vol. 1, Table 23.1
ankle and foot muscles	Vol. 1, Table 23.2

The muscles of the trunk and thigh are shown in Figs 1.12–1.19 in this volume. Tables 1.4a–1.4h show the origin, insertion and action for these muscles.

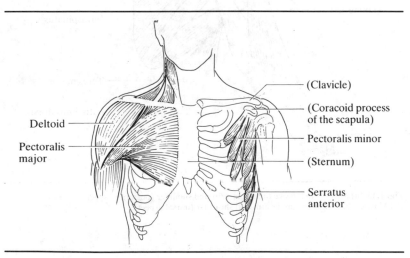

Fig. 1.12 Muscles that move the upper arm and shoulder (anterior aspect)

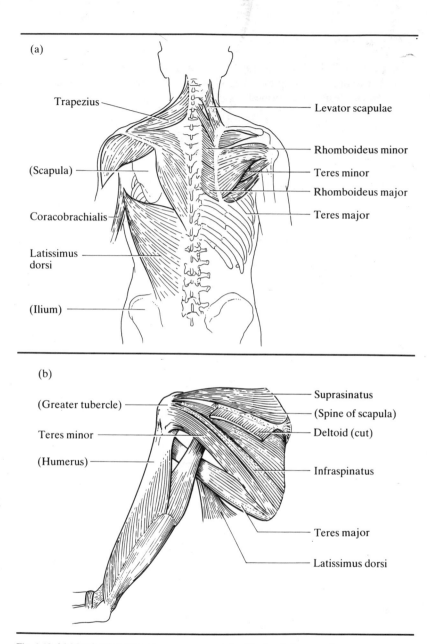

Fig. 1.13 (a) Muscles that move the upper arm and shoulder (posterior aspect)
(b) Muscles that move the upper arm and shoulder (dorsal aspect)

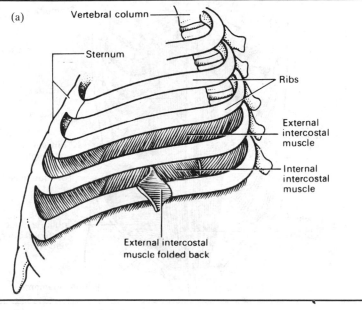

(a)

Vertebral column

Sternum

Ribs

External intercostal muscle

Internal intercostal muscle

External intercostal muscle folded back

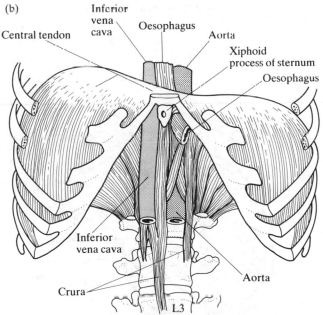

(b)

Central tendon

Inferior vena cava

Oesophagus

Aorta

Xiphoid process of sternum

Oesophagus

Inferior vena cava

Crura

Aorta

L3

Fig. 1.14 (a) The intercostal muscles and the bones of the thorax
(b) Diaphragm

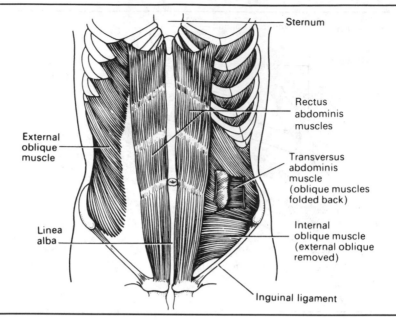

Fig. 1.15 The muscles of the anterior abdominal wall

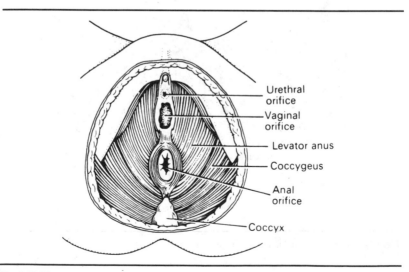

Fig. 1.16 The muscles of the pelvic floor

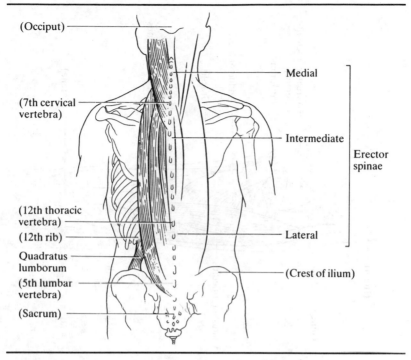

Fig. 1.17 Muscles that move the trunk. Erector spinae and quadratus lomborum

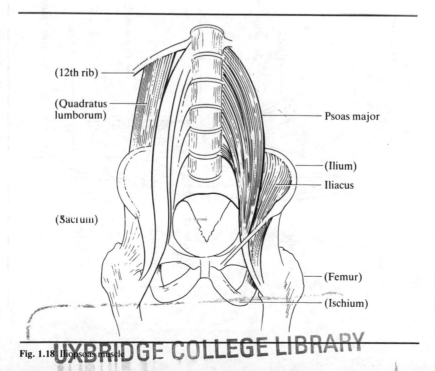

Fig. 1.18 Iliopsoas muscle

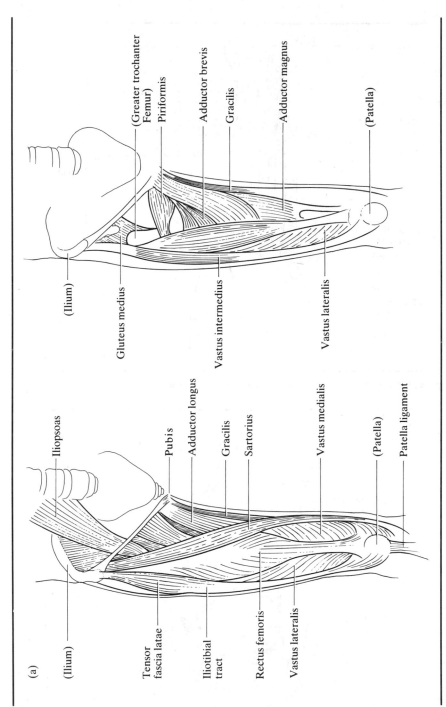

Fig. 1.19 (a) Muscles that move the thigh (anterior aspect)

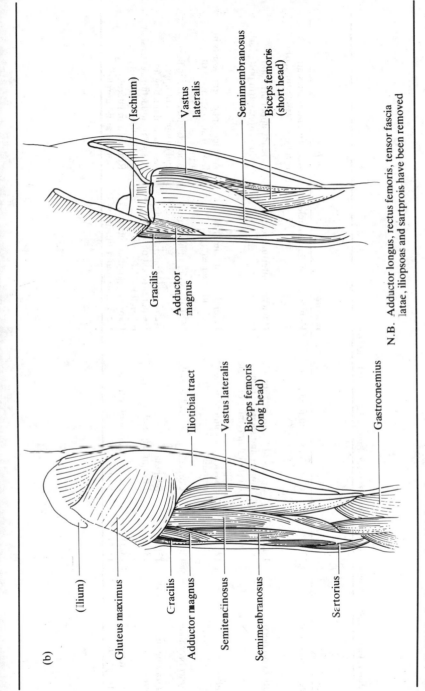

Fig. 1.19 (b) Muscles that move the thigh (posterior aspect)

(b)

(Ilium)
Gluteus maximus
Gracilis
Adductor magnus
Semitendinosus
Semimembranosus
Sartorius

Iliotibial tract
Vastus lateralis
Biceps femoris (long head)
Gastrocnemius

Gracilis
Adductor magnus

(Ischium)
Vastus lateralis
Semimembranosus
Biceps femoris (short head)

N.B. Adductor longus, rectus femoris, tensor fascia latae, iliopsoas and sartorius have been removed

Table 1.4(a) Muscles that move the upper arm (see Figs. 1.12, 1.13(a) and (b))

Name	See Figure No.	Origin	Insertion	Action
Pectoralis major	1.12	Clavicle, sternum, upper 6 costal cartilages	Humerus (greater tubercle)	Adducts and rotates arm medially; draws arm across chest
Latissimus dorsi	1.13(a)	Spines of the lower thoracic, lumbar and sacral vertebrae, crest of ilium, inferior angle of scapula	Humerus (intertubercular groove)	Extends upper arm and adducts upper arm posteriorly
Deltoid	1.12	Clavicle, acromion, spine of scapula	Lateral side of humerus (deltoid tuberosity)	Abducts upper arm, assists in flexion and extension of upper arm
Coracobrachialis	1.13(a)	Coracoid process of scapula	Medial border of humerus	Abducts and assists in flexion and extension of upper arm
Supraspinatus	1.13(b)	Scapula	Humerus (greater tubercle)	Assists in abducting arm
Teres major	1.13(a)	Inferior angle of scapula	Humerus (crest of lesser tubercle)	Assists in adduction, extension and medial rotation of arm
Teres minor	1.13(a)	Lateral margin of scapula	Humerus (greater tubercle)	Rotates arm laterally
Infraspinatus	1.13(b)	Scapula	Humerus (greater tubercle)	Rotates arm laterally

Table 1.4(b) Muscles that move the shoulder (see Figs 1.12 and 1.13(a) and (b))

Name	See Figure No.	Origin	Insertion	Action
Trapezius	1.13(a)	Occipital bone, spinous processes of seventh cervical and all thoracic vertebrae	Clavicle, acromion and spine of scapula	Elevates shoulder, rotates scapula to raise shoulder in abduction of the arm, draws scapula backwards
Pectoralis major	1.12	Clavicle, sternum and upper six ribs	Lateral lip of bicipital groove of humerus	Adducts and flexes arm, medially rotates arm, depresses and protracts the shoulder
Pectoralis minor	1.12	Ribs (second to fifth)	Coracoid process of scapula	Depresses and protracts the scapula
Serratus anterior	1.12	Upper 8 ribs	Vertebral border of scapula	Protracts the scapula and holds it against the ribs, rotates scapula to raise the shoulder in abduction of arm
Rhomboideus major	1.13(a)	Spinous processes of second to fifth thoracic vertebrae	Medial border of scapula	Protracts scapula inwards, retracts and elevates scapula
Rhomboideus minor	1.13(a)	Spinous processes of seventh cervical and first thoracic vertebrae	Medial border of scapula	Retracts the shoulder and elevates the scapula
Levator scapulae	1.13(a)	First to fourth cervical vertebrae	Superior border of scapula	Elevates scapula, rotates scapula inwards

Table 1.4(c) Muscles that move the chest wall (see Figs. 1.14(a) and (b))

Name	See Figure No.	Origin	Insertion	Action
External intercostals (Intercostales externi)	1.14(a)	Inferior border of rib	Superior border of rib	Elevates ribs. Increases size of thorax causing breathing in
Internal intercostals (Intercostales interni)	1.14(a)	Inferior border of rib and costal cartilage	Superior border of rib and costal cartilage below	Possibly depresses ribs when breathing out. Decreases size of thorax
Diaphragm	1.14(b)	Posterior of xiphoid process, costal cartilages, bodies of upper lumbar vertebrae	Central tendon of the diaphragm	Enlarges the thorax causing breathing in

Table 1.4(d) Muscles that move the abdominal wall (see Fig. 1.15)

Name	See Figure No.	Origin	Insertion	Action
External Oblique (Obliquus externus abdominus)	1.15	Lower 8 ribs at costal cartilages	Crest of ilium, linea alba, pubis (by inguinal ligament)	Compresses abdominal viscera, flexes and rotates spinal column
Internal Oblique (Obliquus internus abdominis)	1.15	Iliac crest, fascia, inguinal ligament, lumbodorsal fascia	Lower 3 costal cartilages, linea alba, pubis	Compresses abdominal viscera, flexes and rotates spinal column
Transversus abdominis	1.15	Lower six costal cartilages, iliac crest, inguinal ligament, thoracolumbar fascia	Pubis and linea alba	Compresses abdominal viscera
Rectus abdominis	1.15	Crest of pubis and symphysis of pubis	Xiphoid, fifth, sixth and seventh costal cartilages	Supports abdomen and flexes lumbar vertebrae

N.B. *Inguinal ligament* is a fibrous band from the anterior, superior spine of ilium to the spine of the pubis
Linea alba is the tendinous line from the xiphoid process to the symphysis pubis
Fascia is term for a bend or sheet of tissue investing and connecting muscles.

Table 1.4(e) Muscles of the pelvic floor (see Fig. 1.16)

Name	See Figure No.	Origin	Insertion	Action
Levator ani	1.16	Posterior surface of pubis spine of ischium	Coccyx	Both form floor of pelvic cavity and support pelvic organs
Coccygeus	1.16	Spine of ischium	Coccyx and sacrum	As above

Table 1.4(f) Muscles that move the trunk (see Fig. 1.17)

Name	See Figure No.		Origin	Insertion	Action
Erector spinae (Sacrospinalis)		Lateral	Iliac crest, sacrum, Lower 6 ribs Upper 6 ribs	Lower 6 ribs Upper 6 ribs Fourth to sixth cervical vertebrae	Together they extend the spine and maintain the erect posture of the spine
	1.17	Intermediate	Iliac crest, sacrum Upper 6 thoracic vertebrae	Lower 6 ribs Second to sixth cervical vertebrae	
		Medial	Upper 6 thoracic and last 4 cervical vertebrae	Temporal bone, mastoid process	
Quadratus lumborum (also forms part of posterior abdominal wall)	1.17		Posterior crest of ilium	Twelfth rib	Extend the spine
	1.18		Lower 3 lumbar vertebrae	Transverse processes of the first 4 lumbar vertebrae	

Table 1.4(g) Muscles that move the thigh (see Fig. 1.19 (a) and (b))

Name	See Figure No.	Origin	Insertion	Action
Iliopsoas				
Iliacus	1.18	Iliac fossa of ilium	Lesser trochanter of femur	Flexes thigh
Psoas (major)	1.18	Bodies of twelfth thoracic through to fifth lumbar vertebra	Lesser trochanter of femur	Flexes thigh
Psoas (minor)				
Rectus femoris	1.19(a)	Anterior inferior iliac spine, rim of acetabulum	Tibia (tuberosity), base of patella	Extends leg and flexes thigh
Gluteus maximus	1.19(b)	Posterior aspect of ilium, posterior surface of sacrum and coccyx	Gluteal tuberosity of femur, iliotibial tract	Extends thigh or trunk, rotates thigh laterally
Gluteus medius	1.19(a)	Lateral surface of ilium	Greater trochanter of femur	Abducts and rotates thigh medially, stabilises pelvis on the femur
Gluteus minimus		Lateral surface of ilium	Greater trochanter of femur	Abducts, rotates thigh medially
Tensor fascia latae	1.19(a)	Iliac crest	Tibia through the iliotibial tract	Abducts thigh, flexes and rotates thigh medially
Piriformis	1.19(a)	Ilium and second to fourth sacral vertebrae	Greater trochanter of femur	Rotates thigh laterally, abducts and extends thigh
Adductor brevis	1.19(a)	Body and inferior ramus of pubis	Upper part of linea aspera of femur	Adducts and flexes thigh
Adductor longus	1.19(a)	Body of the pubis	Upper part of linea aspera of femur	Adducts and flexes thigh
Adductor magnus	1.19(a) 1.19(b)	Inferior ramus of pubis, ramus of ischium Ischial tuberosity	Linea aspera of femur Adductor tubercle of femur	Adducts thigh Extends thigh
Gracilis	1.19(b)	Body and inferior ramus of pubis	Medial surface of tibia	Adducts thigh, flexes and adducts leg

N.B. Iliotibial tract is a part of the fascia covering all thigh muscles
Linea aspera is the rough longitudinal line at the back of the femur

Table 1.4(h) Muscles that move the lower leg

Name	See Figure No.	Origin	Insertion	Action
Sartorius	1.19(b)	Anterior superior iliac spines	Tibia (upper medial surface)	Adducts and flexes leg
Quadriceps group:				
Vastus lateralis	1.19(b)	Lateral aspect of femur	Patella	Extends leg
Vastus intermedius	1.19(a)	Anterior and lateral surfaces of femur	Patella	Extends leg
Vastus medialis	1.19(a)	Medial aspect of femur	Patella	Extends leg
Hamstring group				
Biceps femoris	1.19(b)	Long head – tuberosity of ischium Short head – linea aspera of femur	Head of fibula, lateral condyle of tibia	Flexes and rotates leg laterally, extends thigh
Semimembranosus	1.19(b)	Tuberosity of ischium	Lateral condyle of femur, medial condyle of tibia	Flexes leg and extends thigh
Semitendinosus	1.19(b)	Tuberosity of ischium	Tibia (upper medial surface)	Flexes and rotates leg medially, extends thigh

Cavities of the body

Bones and muscles surround and protect four major cavities of the body.

Cranial cavity

This is the hollow space within the cranium which contains the brain, pituitary and pineal glands.

Thoracic cavity (or thorax)

This is the hollow space within the chest which contains the lungs, heart, thymus, oesophagus, trachea, bronchi, aorta, vena cavae and lymphatics.

Abdominal cavity

This is the hollow space between the pelvis and the thorax which comprises the stomach, small intestine, liver, bile ducts, spleen, gall bladder, pancreas, upper part of colon, kidneys, adrenal glands and lymphatics.

Pelvic cavity

The space within the pelvic girdle is continuous with the abdominal cavity and contains the urinary bladder, ureters, pelvic colon, lowest part of the large intestine and rectum and anus. The female pelvis also contains the uterus, the uterine tubes, the ovaries and vagina. The male pelvis contains the prostate gland, seminal vesicles, spermatic cords, deferent ducts and ejaculatory ducts.

Chapter 2

Figure diagnosis

Figure diagnosis is the assessment of the figure. An understanding of body type, posture, postural deformities and defects, figure faults and any other conditions affecting the figure should be known prior to any consultation with the client, as this information provides the basis on which corrective treatments or advice can be given.

Body types

Although people vary in shape and size they usually conform to one of three body types (or somatotypes). For research purposes, Dr William Sheldon's *The Varieties of Human Physique* (1940) provides detailed and specific information on the human physique and its connotations. However, for figure assessment purposes the three somatotypes are as follows.

The endomorph

This type has a roundness of physique and the ability to put on and store fat. There is a predominance of the abdomen over the thorax and of the trunk over the limbs and the overall appearance is usually pear-shaped. The hands and feet may be small and delicate and body movements may be slow and deliberate. Therefore this body type will always have difficulty in maintaining a slim figure (see Fig. 2.1).

The mesomorph

The shape here indicates a predominance of bone and muscle with broad shoulders, a wide muscular neck, a slender waist and well-muscled limbs. This type rarely has weight problems while remaining active (see Fig. 2.1).

The ectomorph

This type is usually very slim with long bones, a flatness of the chest and lacking in muscular bulk. As there is deficiency of the latter, this type may lack strength and stamina and appear lethargic. Often the long, thin trunk is associated with a bent-over posture and also there may be an underweight problem (see Fig. 2.1).

This is a brief summary of body types as few clients will fit exactly into these categories. However, a knowledge of body types makes it easier to appreciate the genetic shape inherited, and is useful in assessing how near or how far the client is from the frame and size of the body type.

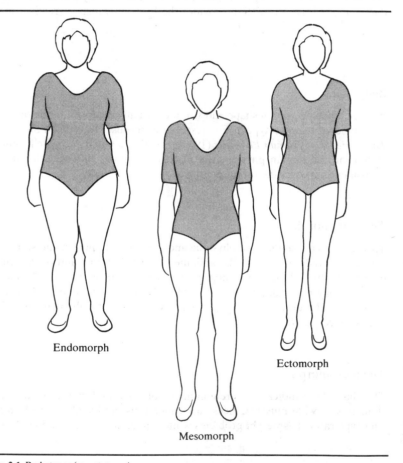

Endomorph

Ectomorph

Mesomorph

Fig. 2.1 Body types (somatotypes)

Posture

Body posture is thought to be good when the maximum efficiency of the body is maintained with the minimum effort. There are three ways in which posture is maintained, i.e. by *postural reflex*, which is the body's response to gravity by co-ordination of the eyes, ears and skin sensation, whereby the brain causes the correct impulses to pass to the muscles which maintain posture; *nervous control*, where posture is maintained by neuro-muscular co-ordination, with impulses passing in the following cycle: muscle – nerve – spinal cord – brain – spinal cord – nerve – muscle; *anti-gravity muscles*, i.e. the muscles which work to overcome gravitational pull and to maintain an erect posture.

Therefore a good posture in a standing position sees the anti-gravity muscles working against the pull of gravity to maintain an erect figure. The centre of gravity of the body is the exact centre of body weight and, in normal posture, the centre of gravity is at the level of the upper sacrum (the second sacral vertebra).

The posture of normal individuals varies considerably and is influenced by such factors as body-build, personality, habits and occupation. Good posture is important as it:

1 keeps muscle action to a minimum thereby saving energy and reducing fatigue;
2 allows a full range of movement;
3 allows full inspiration and expiration movements;
4 reduces the susceptibility of joint injury and back pain;
5 improves physical appearance, whereby the breasts are lifted, the abdomen and buttocks are held in and the head is held erect.

Poor posture wastes energy, increases fatigue and also increases the risk of backache, headache, muscle and ligament strain or joint injury. It may also cause circulatory and digestive disorders, reduce breathing movements and give a poor physical appearance.

A cursory visual assessment of posture can be made when a person is dressed but for a good evaluation the client should wear the minimum of clothing. However, this depends upon the age and temperament of the client and privacy of the area in the salon. When evaluating posture an imaginary line is drawn vertically through the body and this is called the *centre of gravity line*. A plumb line and a tape measure can be useful here and the following points will help to check that the posture of the client conforms to normal posture:

1. From the front or back this line should divide the body into two symmetrical halves (see Fig. 2.2) i.e:

    ● with feet together, the ankles and knees should touch;
    ● the hips should be the same height (a tape measure can be used to measure the height of both hips from the floor);

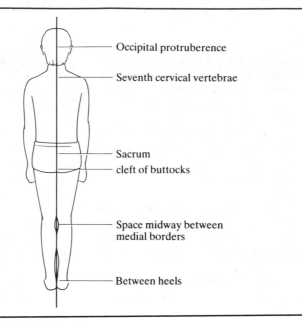

Occipital protruberence

Seventh cervical vertebrae

Sacrum
cleft of buttocks

Space midway between
medial borders

Between heels

Fig. 2.2 Lateral gravity line

- the shoulders should be level (this can be checked by measuring the height to the acromion process).
2. The sternum and vertebral column should run down the centre of the body in line with the centre-of-gravity line. A plumb line falling midway between the heels bisects the cleft of the buttocks, sacrum, seventh cervical vertebra and occipital protuberance. Although slight deviations are common, irregularities in symmetry beyond a minor degree should be noted.
3. The head should be erect, i.e. not tilted to one side.
4. From the sides (see Fig. 2.3) this line should pass through the:
   - foot – anterior to the lateral malleolus of the fibula;
   - knee – posterior to the patella;
   - hip – through greater trochanter of femur;
   - shoulder – centre of acromion process;
   - head – through the ear lobe (or mastoid process).

Postural defects

Postural defects may be considered as variations from the accepted normal posture and many of these can be corrected by active, muscular effort by the

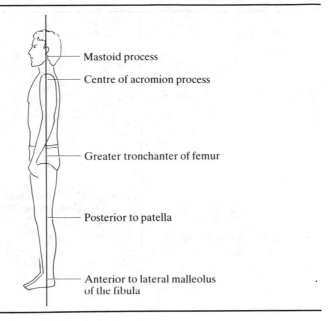

Mastoid process

Centre of acromion process

Greater tronchanter of femur

Posterior to patella

Anterior to lateral malleolus
of the fibula

Fig. 2.3 Anteroposterior gravity line

client. However, there are some conditions, especially of the spine, that may be the result of injury, an acquired disease or a congenital disorder or disease which never develops from poor posture. Some of these diseases or deformities can be recognised and are explained in 1–6 (below).

1. Lumbar lordosis

This is abnormally increased posterior concavity in the curvature of the lumbar spine where the pelvis tilts forward and the spine follows its movement. As the back is hollow, the abdomen and buttocks protrude and the knees may be hyperextended (see Fig. 2.4).

2. Kyphosis

This is an abnormally increased posterior convexity in the curvature of the thoracic spine as viewed from the side. The back appears round as the shoulders point forward. The ear lobe is behind the tip of the shoulder and if the head moves forward the chin usually protrudes. Often there is a tightness of the pectoral muscles. Where there is a severe degree of kyphosis and lordosis this is known as kypholordosis (see Fig. 2.5).

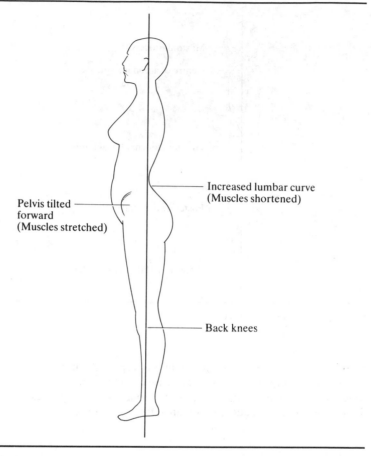

Pelvis tilted
forward
(Muscles stretched)

Increased lumbar curve
(Muscles shortened)

Back knees

Fig. 2.4 Lordosis

3. Structural scoliosis

This is the lateral curvature of the vertebral column which may be to the right or left side. The first visible signs are likely to be unevenness of the hips and shoulders or curvature of the spine and sometimes there is a deformity of the rib cage (see also postural scoliosis in (Fig. 2.6 (a)).

4. Pes planus (flat feet)

The medial longitudinal arch looks flat and the medial border of the foot is convex. If the condition is structural the deformity persists.

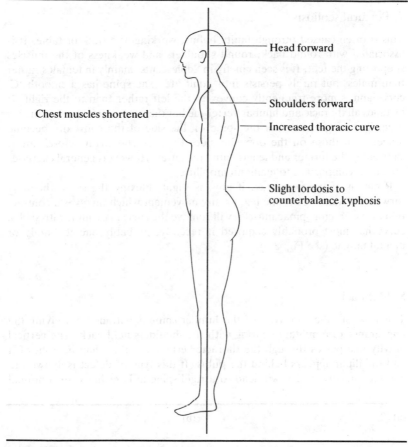

Head forward

Shoulders forward

Increased thoracic curve

Chest muscles shortened

Slight lordosis to
counterbalance kyphosis

Fig. 2.5 Kyphosis

5. Genus valgum (knock knees)

This is an inward curving of the knees which is usually caused by irregular
bone growth or by weak ligaments. The ankles do not touch each other when
the legs are together and the feet are pointing forward.

6. Genus varum (bandy or bow legs)

This is a deformity in which the space between the knees is abnormally large,
again usually caused by irregular bone growth where the shafts of the femur,
tibia and fibular are turned outwards.

7. Postural scoliosis

This is often caused through faulty habits, working at a desk or table. It is associated with round back, round shoulders and weakness of the muscles supporting the feet. It is seen chiefly in adolescents, mainly in females rather than males, but rarely persists into adult life. The spine has a smooth 'C' curve and is more frequently convex to the left rather than to the right. It includes all thoracic and lumbar vertebrae but there is no deformity of the rib cage. The long muscles of the spine on the side of the convexity become longer than those on the opposite side. Exercise should therefore aim at shortening the former and lengthening the latter. However, general exercises are equally important to maintain mobility.

Rotation of the vertebrae, if any, is slight. Flexing the spine, bending forward or standing on one leg, or any movement which involves a contraction of the erector spinae muscle, will remove the curve. An adult with such a curve has most probably acquired it recently, probably due to bodily or mental fatigue (see Fig. 2.6).

8. Flat back

This is where the concavity of the lumbar spine is flattened out giving the appearance of a military bearing with the shoulders held back. The vertical gravity line passes through the thoracic vertebrae rather than in front of it and the ilium appears behind the pubis. If this type of defect is allowed to continue uncorrected it will lead to a rigid spine in later life with continual

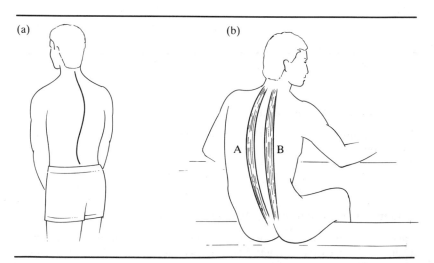

Fig. 2.6 (a) Postural scoliosis
(b) Faulty sitting position with
A lengthened long and spinal muscles
B shortened long spinal muscles

backache. The client should be given mobility exercises for the spine and the legs, as a flat back is often associated with congenital shortening of the hamstring muscles (see Fig. 2.7).

9. Round shoulders

This seldom exists as a single defect. It often happens when the muscles which link the scapulae with the spine allow the scapulae to slip forward and downward due to the action of gravity. The condition may simply be attributed to poor posture or a lack of adipose tissue to pad and round out the contours. Continual forward positioning of the head can often lead to a condition known as *Dowager's hump* and this is where fatty deposits accumulate over the base of the neck and top of the spine. Also associated with

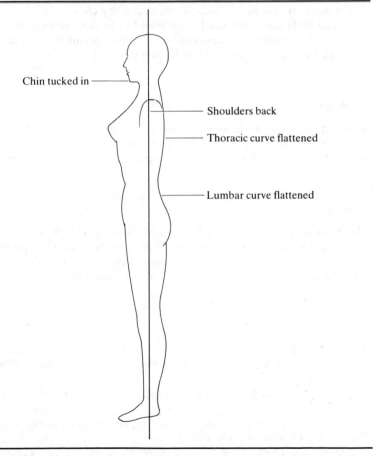

Chin tucked in

Shoulders back

Thoracic curve flattened

Lumbar curve flattened

Fig. 2.7 Flat back

round shoulders are shortened pectoral muscles, a hollow chest and inflexibi-
lity of the rib cage which can cause breathing to be affected. Simple exercises
to improve the condition should be given, i.e. grasping the hands behind the
head and pushing the elbows backwards and showing the client deep breathing exercises to create movement of the rib cage.

Most defects can be improved with suitable exercises but in some cases
where there is considerable deviation medical opinion should be sought.

Figure faults

1. Head

(a) *Head thrust* exists where the centre of the ear is not in alignment with the
centre of the shoulder. This is a very common fault where the head is
brought forward by reading, typing, computing etc.
(b) *Head tilt* is where the head is inclined to one side. Both faults can be
corrected by similar exercises which involve stretching the muscles of the
neck by rotation of the head and tilting the head from side to side.

2. Shoulders

Shoulder levels vary in almost everyone and these variations are often caused
by carrying heavy articles incorrectly. Drooping shoulders are a prelude to
round shoulders and the client should be made aware of good posture.

3. Arms

These can vary from the thin, scrawny arm with loose crêpey skin, as seen in
the elderly or underweight clients, to the plump arm with fatty deposits. The
latter is often associated with the overweight client and concentrated treatments and exercises are needed to make an improvement.

4. Breasts

The sternum and rib cage are involved in the way the breasts are positioned
on the chest wall; therefore any chest deformity, i.e. pigeon chest (a projecting sternum) or hollow (concave) chest, should be observed.

Breasts do not contain muscular tissue but are supported by the suspensory
ligaments of Cooper which are fibrous tissues and these connect with the
fascia of the chest wall and with the subcutaneous tissues of the skin. It is
these ligaments which uphold and hold forward the breasts. They act against
gravity to give support. The size and shape of the breasts are usually deter-

mined by genetic factors. The overall size and shape of the client's build should be taken into consideration as the quantity of surface fat present on the body alters the breast size and shape.

Thin people often have small underdeveloped breasts due to lack of adipose tissue. Underdeveloped breasts can also be caused by muscle weakness. The pectoral muscles cannot contract and the trapezius muscles expand giving the client a round-shouldered appearance.

You will certainly have clients with sagging breasts and these are due in the main to:

● heavy breasts;
● lack of good support;
● badly fitting bra;
● poor posture;
● muscle tone;
● dieting;
● age (breasts atrophy with age and there is a loss of tissue).

Breast sag can be measured by holding a pencil underneath the breast. If the pencil stays in place, there is breast sag. Exercise will help medium sag and help maintain a firm bust.

Other physical features to be taken into account are whether there are lumps present that move, or one breast is larger than the other, or if there is excessive hair growth in the area and whether inverted nipples are present.

5. Waist and abdomen

Poor muscle tone and excess adipose tissue will result in a protrusion of the abdominal wall and a thickening of the waist. Any operations in this area will have an adverse effect on muscular strength. The weight carried in front during pregnancy often causes the body's balance to be affected and a pelvic tilt may be present.

6. Buttocks

These are usually an area where fatty deposits settle easily – often an occupational hazard of sedentary workers. The shape of the buttocks should be observed, to note whether the area is round and firm or whether there are fat deposits over the deep gluteal fascia covering the buttocks and thighs. It is a common figure problem which may indicate either that a weight loss is needed or simply a reduction in inches is required.

7. Legs

The shape of the legs generally relate to the body type or the genetic shape inherited. Muscular legs are usually developed by sport (see Cellulite, below). The circulation of the legs is important; look for oedema (an excessive accumulation of serous fluid in the tissues) especially in the ankles and a note should be made for thread or varicose veins as these restrict certain treatments.

8. Feet

As feet are subjected to a great deal of strain, foot disorders occur. One of the most common disorders and one which can result in pain when standing or walking is 'flat feet'. This is caused by the flattening of the medial longitudinal arch. In the healthy foot, the arches are supported by muscles but when these fail to support the arch or become weak the arch is only supported by strong ligaments. As the ligaments become strained, the arch flattens. When observing the feet also note if there are bunions, corns or hammer toes present as these can affect the normal posture.

Other conditions affecting the figure

Obesity

Obesity is an excessive accumulation of fat in the body and is apparent when anyone is 10 per cent over the ideal figure weight. There are various forms of obesity, i.e:

● nervous obesity, which usually affects women and children under stress;
● endocrine obesity, which comes from under-secretion of the thyroid gland (see Chap. 3), and this hypothyroidism causes slow metabolism, resulting in too much cellular fluid;
● hereditary obesity is, as the name implies, a genetic factor;
● habit obesity, which is self-explanatory and usually a result of boredom;
● drug obesity, which can occur when a client has to take a drug which slows down the metabolism.

Being overweight can affect physical and mental health. Too many extra pounds can put a strain on the body and can eventually shorten the span of life. Obesity, being unattractive, may create psychological problems, and the subject is further analysed in Chapter 6.

Cellulite

Cellulite is not a word or condition recognised by the medical profession. as far as they are concerned fat is fat! In the beauty-therapy field we regard cellulite as an amassed number of cells which contain waste products and toxins and if the latter are left over after normal metabolism (see Chap. 6) they stagnate and cause retention of water in and around the fat cells.

Cellulite frequently plagues women of normal weight and generally fails to respond to diet and exercise and is always localised. Soft cellulite gives the skin the appearance of orange peel as it is pitted and, when pinched, looks dimpled and tiny nodules can be felt underneath which roll like grains of rice under pressure from the thumb. It has complex links with the female hormonal cycle and can appear at puberty, during pregnancy, from ten to two days prior to menstruation or at the onset of the menopause.

It can also be caused by stress or by certain drugs, i.e. tranquillisers, sleeping pills and anti-depressants. These drugs, taken over a long period, create an accumulation of toxic waste in the system. Therefore the aim must be to improve the circulation of the areas affected and generally invigorate and tone all the systems of the body.

The main areas requiring treatment are the tricep muscles of the arms, the latissimus dorsi muscles of the middle back, the rectus abdominis, external and internal oblique, and transverse abdominis muscles of the abdomen, the tensor fascia latae muscles of the thigh and the glutei of the buttocks.

Hard cellulite is usually found in dancers, athletes and older women. If it has been built up over a long time, the surface skin may be smooth but there may be lumpy areas. The tissues may be painful, liable to bruising and highly inflexible. If the skin has been over-stretched there may be light scarring caused through the breaking down of the elastin and collagen fibres. Hard cellulite needs frequent, long-term treatment to decongest the tissues, break up fatty deposits, restore tone and elasticity, re-establish healthy circulation and correct lymphatic drainage. It is often called *trapped fat* as the fatty tissue is present between the muscle fibres.

Fluid retention

This can cause bloating of the tissues or oedema and is one of the reasons for the formation of cellulite. As the endocrine glands are primarily responsible for the normal hormonal balance in the body, (see Chap. 3) any imbalance will result in fluid retention.

Cardiac oedema shows swelling of the ankles and feet. The skin is pale and soft but there is no tenderness of the swollen tissues.

Menstrual oedema often occurs during the week preceding menstruation and is often accompanied with tension in the breasts, lower abdominal fullness, nervous irritability and a frontal headache.

Gravitational oedema, i.e. swollen legs or hands, are often the result of a client's standing all day or simply drinking numerous cups of coffee or tea. It can also be due to excessive salt in the diet, an underactive kidney or to a congenital defect.

Consultation techniques

A consultation with the client provides the therapist with the opportunity to obtain certain information to help determine the treatment plan. Remember that the client is seeking advice because of a desire to improve appearance, to improve the quality of life or ease stress or tension. It is important to create a sympathetic and professional atmosphere whereby a rapport between the therapist and client can develop which obviously increases the client's confidence and co-operation. Mentally observe the overall shape of the client from the moment he or she enters the salon. Note posture, figure shape and size, as these form part of the *visual assessment*.

During an initial consultation record your client's personal details, i.e. full name, address, telephone number, date of birth (or age), client's doctor's name, address and telephone number (if known). Try to obtain information on the client's life style, i.e. active or inactive; are hobbies, sports or exercise undertaken? Check gynaecological history and number and ages of children (if female), allergies, and note any medication currently being taken (see Fig. 2.8).

Clients are often forgetful or reluctant to admit to taking tablets, pills or drugs. This information is vital to your assessment and treatment plan. It has been known for a client to collapse in a sauna or steam cabinet after taking a heavy dose of sleeping tablets or tranquillisers. If a client has had several courses of antibiotics, tiredness and exhaustion may linger for several weeks and be a contra-indication to general heat treatments and the use of the sunbed.

Check medical background for any muscular disorder, recent operations or heart disorders etc., which would preclude electrical treatment or strenuous exercises. If voluntary exercise is inadvisable because of illness or physical condition, the client's doctor should be consulted before embarking on a course of treatments. Electronic stimulation should not be used on any part of the body where the skin, superficial fascia or muscle are in any way inflamed or swollen through disease or injury.

Check skin for rashes, scratches etc. and small breaks should be covered with adhesive before treatments.

Once a rapport has been created and the reason for the client's visit to the salon has been established, weight and accurate measurements can be taken in a private cubicle or room. Many clients may find this embarrassing if they are not approached in a professional manner. Initially, a client who is extremely shy may only wish to be weighed, and skilful client handling will be required before the figure diagnosis chart (or card) can be completed (see Fig. 2.8).

Procedure for figure diagnosis

Request the client to undress. Remember many women may prefer to retain their bra and pants. However, large-boned or restricting bras should be

Figure Diagnosis Chart (or card printed both sides)

Name: ....

Address: ....

....

Telephone No: ....

Date of birth: ....

Occupation: ....

Hobbies: ....

Female: ....

  Number of pregnancies: ....

  Date of last pregnancy: ....

Other: ....

....

Dr. name: ....

Address: ....

....

Telephone No: ....

Medical history: ....

....

....

Medication: ....

....

....

Allergies: ....

....

Measurements:

Height: .... Weight: ....

Frame size: ....

Ideal weight: ....

Posture: ....

Contra-indications: ....

....

....

	Date: ...		Date: ...		Type of fat	Muscle tone
Upper arm	R:	L:	R:	L:		
Wrist	R:	L:	R:	L:		
Chest or bust						
Rib cage						
Waist						
Upper abdomen						
Lower abdomen						
Buttocks						
Upper thigh	R:	L:	R:	L:		
Mid thigh	R:	L:	R:	L:		
Above knee	R:	L:	R:	L:		
Below knee	R:	L:	R:	L:		
Ankle	R:	L:	R:	L:		

Fig. 2.8 Figure diagnosis chart

removed if they cover too much of the abdomen, or if specific advice is required on breast and shoulder problems. Men should wear underpants.

1. Measure height and weight

The client is then weighed once a week, or more frequently if a diet is being followed. There can be a weight gain during the day of up to 3 lb (1.36 kg) from food and liquid consumed. Therefore it is preferable to weigh the client at the same time on each visit to the salon. Compare weight against weight tables detailed in Table 2.1(a) for women and Table 2.1(b) for men. If the client is between 10 lb (4.54 kg) and 15 lb (6.80 kg) overweight or underweight, ask a few questions, i.e. are parents or family overweight/underweight, recent marriage, date of birth of the last child, change of job, stress, and length of time since overweight/underweight, i.e. always or recent?

2. Observation of the client

Is he or she nervous or placid, slow or quick in movement. Have a full-length mirror available and scrutinize the client from all sides. It is better for the client not to view him/herself in the mirror until your scrutiny is over, otherwise abdominal muscles will be pulled in and posture will be corrected!

3. Decide on type of body physique and check posture

Make notes on any deviation from normal posture as this will affect treatments and suggested exercise programme. To determine an average frame weight for the client, measure the wrist (see Table 2.2(a)). Calculations can then be made to give average figure measurements (see Table 2.2(b)).

4. Measure the client

Do this carefully with a wide tape measure, as follows.

Upper arms
Measure 2–3 in (5–8 cm) down from the axillae. Is the muscle tone firm or slack, are the arms too thin or fat?

Chest   For the male, this is relatively easy. Ensure the tape is flat and straight at the back and measure over the nipples. Breasts or mammary glands exist in the male in a rudimentary form. Enlargement of the breasts in the male is called gynecomastia and is not an uncommon occurrence during adolescence.

Table 2.1 (a) Average weights for women

Height		Small frame	Medium frame	Large frame
4ft 8in	st lb	6.2 – 6.7	6.6 – 7.3	7.0 – 8.1
1.42m	lb	86 – 93	90 – 101	98 – 113
	kg	39.04 – 42.22	40.86 – 45.85	44.49 – 51.30
4ft 9in	st lb	6.4 – 6.10	6.7 – 7.6	7.4 – 8.4
1.45m	lb	88 – 94	91 – 104	102 – 116
	kg	39.95 – 42.68	41.31 – 47.22	46.31 – 52.66
4ft 10in	st lb	6.6 – 7.0	6.12 – 7.9	7.7 – 8.8
1.47m	lb	90 – 98	96 – 107	105 – 120
	kg	40.86 – 44.49	43.58 – 48.58	47.67 – 54.48
4ft 11in	st lb	7.6 – 7.13	7.12 – 8.6	8.5 – 9.1
1.50m	lb	104 – 111	110 – 118	111 – 127
	kg	47.2 – 50.4	49.9 – 53.6	50.4 – 57.66
5ft	st lb	7.7 – 8.1	8.0 – 8.8	8.7 – 9.3
1.52m	lb	105 – 113	112 – 120	119 – 129
	kg	47.67 – 51.30	50.85 – 54.48	54.03 – 58.57
5ft 1in	st lb	7.9 – 8.3	8.2 – 8.10	8 10 – 9.5
1.55,	lb	107 – 115	114 – 122	122 – 131
	kg	48.58 – 52.21	51.76 – 55.39	55.39 – 59.47
5ft 2in	st lb	7.12 – 8.6	8.5 – 8.13	8.12 – 9.9
1.57m	lb	110 – 118	117 – 125	124 – 135
	kg	49.94 – 53.57	53.12 – 56.75	53.30 – 61.29
5ft 3in	st lb	8.1 – 8.9	8.8 – 9.2	9.1 – 9.12
1.60m	lb	113 – 121	120 – 128	127 – 138
	kg	51.30 – 54.93	54.48 – 58.12	57.66 – 62.65
5ft 4in	st lb	8.4 – 8.13	8.12 – 9.6	9.5 – 10.2
1.63m	lb	116 – 125	124 – 132	131 – 142
	kg	52.66 – 56.75	56.30 – 59.02	59.47 – 64.47
5ft 5in	st lb	8.7 – 9.2	9.1 – 9.9	9.7 – 10.5
1.65m	lb	119 – 128	127 – 135	133 – 145
	kg	54.03 – 58.11	57.66 – 61.29	60.38 – 65.83
5ft 6in	st lb	8.11 – 9.6	9.4 – 10.0	9.12 – 10.10
1.68m	lb	123 – 132	130 – 140	138 – 150
	kg	55.84 – 59.93	59.02 – 63.56	62.65 – 68.10
5ft 7in	st lb	9.0 – 9.10	9.8 – 10.4	10 2 – 11.0
1.70m	lb	126 – 136	134 – 144	142 – 154
	kg	57.20 – 61.74	60.84 – 65.38	64.47 – 69.92
5ft 8in	st lb	9.3 – 9.13	9.11 – 10.7	10.5 – 11.4
1.73m	lb	129 – 139	137 – 147	145 – 158
	kg	58.57 – 63.11	62.20 – 66.74	65.83 – 71.73
5ft 9in	st lb	9.7 – 10.3	10.1 – 10.11	10.9 – 11.8
1.75m	lb	133 – 143	141 – 151	149 – 162
	kg	60.38 – 64.92	64.01 – 68.55	67.65 – 73.55
5ft 10in	st lb	9.10 – 10.7	10.5 – 11.1	10.12 – 11.12
1.78m	lb	136 – 147	145 – 155	152 – 166
	kg	61.74 – 66.74	65.83 – 70.37	69.00 – 75.36
5 ft 11in	st lb	9.13 – 10.10	10.8 – 11.4	11.1 – 12.1
1.80m	lb	139 – 150	148 – 158	155 – 169
	kg	63.11 – 68.10	67.19 – 71.73	70.37 – 76.73

Table 2.1 (b)   Average weights for men

Height		Small frame	Medium frame	Large frame
5ft 1in	st lb	8.1 – 8.7	8.7 – 9.0	9.4 – 9.10
1.55in	lb	113 – 119	119 – 126	130 – 136
	kg	51.30 – 54.03	54.03 – 57.20	59.02 – 61.74
5ft 2in	st lb	8.4 – 8.10	8.11 – 9.4	9.7 – 9.11
1.57m	lb	116 – 122	123 – 130	133 – 137
	kg	52.66 – 55.39	55.84 – 59.02	60.38 – 62.20
5ft 3in	st lb	8.7 – 9.0	9.1 – 9.8	9.11 – 10.4
1.60m	lb	119 – 126	127 – 134	137 – 144
	kg	54.03 – 57.20	57.66 – 60.84	62.20 – 65.38
5ft 4in	st lb	8.10 – 9.4	9.3 – 9.11	9.12 – 10.6
1.63m	lb	122 – 130	129 – 137	138 – 146
	kg	55.39 – 59.02	58.57 – 62.20	62.65 – 66.28
5ft 5in	st lb	8.12 – 9.6	9.6 – 10.2	10.3 – 10.11
1.65m	lb	124 – 132	132 – 142	143 – 151
	kg	56.30 – 59.93	59.93 – 64.47	64.92 – 68.55
5ft 6in	st lb	9.2 – 9.12	9.10 – 10.6	10.8 – 11.4
1.68m	lb	128 – 138	136 – 146	148 – 158
	kg	58.11 – 62.65	61.74 – 66.28	67.19 – 71.73
5ft 7in	st lb	9.7 – 10.2	10.0 – 10.9	10.12 – 11.7
1.70m	lb	133 – 142	140 – 149	152 – 161
	kg	60.38 – 64.47	63.56 – 67.65	69.10 – 73.09
5ft 8in	st lb	9.8 – 10.5	10.5 – 11.0	11.3 – 11.12
1.73m	lb	134 – 145	145 – 154	157 – 166
	kg	60.84 – 65.83	65.83 – 69.92	71.28 – 75.36
5ft 9in	st lb	10.1 – 10.11	10.9 – 11.3	11.6 – 12.0
1.75m	lb	141 – 151	149 – 157	160 – 168
	kg	64.01 – 68.55	67.65 – 71.28	72.64 – 76.27
5ft 10in	st lb	10.4 – 11.1	10.13 – 11.9	11.13 – 12.7
1.78m	lb	144 – 155	153 – 163	167 – 175
	kg	65.38 – 70.37	69.46 – 74.00	75.82 – 79.45
5ft 11in	st lb	10.9 – 11.5	11.4 – 12.0	12.2 – 12.12
1.80m	lb	149 – 159	158 – 168	170 – 180
	kg	67.65 – 72.19	71.73 – 76.27	77.18 – 81.72
6ft	st lb	10.13 – 11.9	11.8 – 12.4	12.6 – 13.2
1.83m	lb	153 – 163	162 – 172	174 – 184
	kg	69.46 – 74.00	73.55 – 78.09	79.00 – 83.54
6ft 1in	st lb	11.3 – 11.12	11.13 – 12.8	12.13 – 13.6
1.85m	lb	157 – 166	167 – 176	181 – 188
	kg	71.28 – 75.36	75.82 – 79.90	82.17 – 85.35
6ft 2in	st lb	11.7 – 12.2	12.4 – 13.0	13.2 – 13.12
1.88m	lb	161 – 170	172 – 182	184 – 194
	kg	73.09 – 77.18	78.09 – 82.63	83.54 – 88.08
6ft 3in	st lb	11.13 – 12.7	12.9 – 13.5	13.7 – 14.3
1.90m	lb	167 – 175	177 – 187	189 – 199
	kg	75.82 – 7 9.45	80.36 – 84.90	85.81 – 90.35

Breast diagnosis
For the female this should not be undertaken in isolation to the rest of the
body. Measurements should be taken of the breasts over the nipples, the
waist, and upper and lower hips to ascertain if these parts of the body are in

Table 2.2 (a)   Wrist measurements used as a guide to average frame weight

Wrist	Height	Frame
Less than 5½in 13.97cm	4ft 11in – 5ft 2in 1.50m – 1.57m	Very small
Less than 6in 15.24cm	5ft 3in – 5ft 4in 1.60m – 1.63m	Small
Less than 6¼in 15.88cm	5ft 5in – 5ft 11in 1.65m – 1.80m	Small/medium
5½in to 5¾in 13.97 to 14.60cm	4ft 11in – 5ft 2in 1.50m – 1.57m	Small/medium
6in to 6¼in 15.24 to 15.88cm	5ft 3in – 5ft 4in 1.60m – 1.63m	Medium
6¼in to 6½in 15.88cm to 16.51cm	5ft 5in – 5ft 11in 1.65m – 1.80m	Medium/large
More than 5¾in 14.60cm	4ft 11in – 5ft 2in 1.50m – 1.57m	Medium/large
More than 6¼in 15.88cm	5ft 3in – 5ft 4in 1.60m – 1.63m	Large
More than 6½in 16.51cm	5ft 5in – 5ft 11in 1.65m – 1.80m	Very large

Table 2.2 (b)   An example of average figure measurements for a medium frame 5ft 3in to 5ft 4in or 1.60m to 1.63m.

6in Wrist – 15.24cm

Bust 6in or 15.24cm × 6	=	36in or 91.44cm
Waist 6in or 15.24cm × 6	=	24in or 60.96cm
Hips 6in or 15.24cm × 6¼	=	37½in or 95.25cm
Thighs 6in or 15.24cm × 3⅓	=	20in or 50.75cm
Ankles 6in or 15.24cm × 1⅓	=	8in or 20.27cm

proportion. Check the position of the breasts on the chest wall and compare the size of them in relation to the rest of the body and to each other. Observe the nipples, i.e. puffy areolae are a sign of an underdeveloped bust; a retraction of the nipples is often caused by under active glands or could have serious medical implications and, without alarming the client, she should be referred to her own doctor. Also note if there is any weeping from the nipple itself. Hypertrophy of the breasts, abnormal enlargement of the breasts, is often a symptom of an endocrine disorder.

Another method to check the bust for muscle tone or the degree of bust sag present, is to request the client to lie on the couch, raise one hand above the head horizontally and determine the measurement between that breast and the one on the other side. If the nipple does not move, there is 100 per cent sag, if it moves at least 2 in (5 cm) there is good muscle tone present. However, if there is only 1 in (2.5 cm) variation there is still some muscle tone, and treatment with exercise and the use of the faradic current on the pectoral muscles will improve the bust.

Factors which need to be taken into consideration are age, menopause, childbirth and sudden loss of weight which shows in breasts by stretch marks and wrinkling of the skin due to loss of adipose tissue.

Abdomen

To check for muscle tone request the client to inhale and 'pull in' the stomach (to separate muscle from fat) as hard as possible to flatten the abdominal wall and hold for a few seconds. If the rectus abdominis and the external oblique muscles are in good muscle tone the abdominal wall may flatten until it is almost concave. Muscles which are stretched will not affect a full contraction easily and will be unable to sustain a tetanic (i.e. muscles acting through nervous control) contraction for any length of time. Any fatty deposits can be felt with the fingers and are clearly visible when the muscles are contracted.

There is another test which can be given to test the strength of abdominal muscles, but this should not be given if there is any weakness in the lumbar area. Have the client lie in a supine (lying on the back) position on the floor and raise both legs about 6 in (15.5 cm) above the floor. One leg should be lifted as high as possible and then with both legs the client should attempt a 'walking' movement without either leg touching the floor. If 12–24 strides can be accomplished the muscles are fairly strong but less than 12 strides indicates poor muscle tone.

Buttocks and backs of thighs

Measurements taken when measuring the breast should have been over the widest part of the buttocks and below the gluteal fold. Always ensure that the tape measure is flat and straight. Check that the hips are horizontally level.

To test the strength of the gluteal muscles, request the client to pretend that there is a penny between the buttocks and to hold this imaginary penny there as tightly as possible. With good muscle tone the gluteus maximus will contract and lift strongly and the muscles of the thigh may also contract slightly. Contraction will not be possible if there is poor muscle tone and lack of co-ordination of the glutei.

Muscle strength in the pelvic area can also be assessed by a simple exercise. Request the client to stand with feet 12 in (35 cm) apart and, with the knees bent, to extend the arms slowly in front of the body but at the same time to tilt the pelvis backwards without moving the legs or upper part of the body. Then ask the client to swing the arms slowly behind and at the same time tilt the pelvis forward. The muscles at the back of the thigh (i.e. biceps femoris, semitendinosus, semimembranosus and glutei) and front of the thigh (i.e. rectus femoris) should contract. If the movements are performed easily and the client can keep the pelvis tilting in a smooth arc with firm control, the muscle tone is likely to be good. On the other hand, if the movements are difficult to achieve, muscle tone is poor, probably from lack of use.

Thighs

Take two measurements at the top of both thighs and midway to the knees. It is rare to find both thighs having the exact same measurements as clients usually have a habit of increasing muscle bulk by standing, or partaking in sporting activities, where one leg is used more than the other. Check for the amount of adipose tissue present and note whether the muscle tone is poor or good.

Legs

Measurements should be taken above and below the knees. Often there are pads of soft fatty tissue on the inside of the knees. Note if the knees have any abnormality, hyper-extended knees (back knees) or those described in *Postural defects* (5 and 6, see p. 43). Check the legs for varicose or thread veins.

Ankles and feet

Measurement of the ankle should be taken if oedema exists. Check the feet for pes planus or for any other foot pronation, i.e. if the line of the Achilles tendon slants medially, this deviation involves eversion of the calcaneus. Also note if toes are misaligned, or if corns or bunions present.

For maximum accuracy subsequent measurements should be taken by the same therapist.

The answers that the client gives to the questions asked and commonsense observation by the therapist provide pointers to aid in determining the prime factors causing the figure problem. A poor figure and/or bulky misshapen body may be due to one or several of the following:

● poor posture;
● fat deposits;
● overweight;
● slack and atrophied musculature;
● overdeveloped musculature;
● excess water retention.

Each of these requires different treatment; therefore a thorough figure diagnosis must be carried out before beginning any treatment.

Assessment and treatment plan

The assessment made by the beauty therapist during a consultation will form the basis of all future contact with the client. It is important that the client understands the advice given and, because this is not always absorbed by the client at the first consultation, it should be repeated during a subsequent visit. Any contra indication to beauty-therapy treatment is based on the evaluation of the information obtained and any apparent symptoms or signs. A full explanation must be given to the client as to why a certain treatment may not be performed and the therapist should be aware of the alternatives available.

The treatment plan requires careful discussion with the client and should include salon treatments, techniques and products and advice on home treat-

Recommended salon treatments/exercise/diet for:-

Name: ....

Address: ....
....

Salon treatments:	Dates given	Results (if any)
Type:	....	....
....	....	....
....	....	....
....	....	....

Excercise:	Dates given	Muscle tone improvement
Type:	....	....
....	....	....
....	....	....
....	....	....

Diet:	Dates checked	Weight loss or gain
Type:	....	....
No. of calories	....	....
	....	....
	....	....

Recommended home products/exercise/diet

Products: ....
....

Exercise:	Date given:
Type:	....
....	....
....	....

Diet:

Type:	....
Number of calories:	....
....	....

Other: ....
....

Fig. 2.9 Treatment chart

ments and products. Fig. 2.9 is a suggested form or card for record purposes which can be attached to the figure diagnosis chart.

The client will want to know the length of time it will take to complete a series of treatments, how many visits are required to the salon and what length of interval can be left between treatments and, finally, and often the most important, the cost. This should be explained carefully as the treatment plan must provide optimum improvement, satisfaction and benefit.

Chapter 3

The communication systems

The nervous system and the endocrine systems together fulfil a vital function for the body – communication. They are complicated systems and for the beauty therapist only the basic knowledge is required.

The nervous system

The nervous system of the body is a system of cells that forms a communication system between receptors, which sense changes in the environment, and effectors, which produce response to stimuli.

It has two main divisions, dependent upon each other, which are as follows:

● the central nervous system (CNS) consisting of the brain and the spinal cord; and
● the peripheral nervous system (PNS) which consists of 31 pairs of spinal nerves, 12 pairs of cranial nerves and the autonomic system which is divided into two parts, sympathetic and parasympathetic.

Nervous tissue

Nervous tissue consists of nerve cells called *neurones* which are supported by a type of connective tissue known as *neuroglia*. There are three types of neurone, i.e. multipolar, bipolar and unipolar (as explained in Vol. 1, Chap. 2). Each neurone consists of:

1 *a cell body* containing the cell nucleus and cytoplasm, which are concerned with the nutrition of the cell;
2 two types of *nerve fibres* which are threadlike extensions of the cell body and called *dendrites* and *axons*.

Nerve fibres possess the power of conductivity and excitability. They are capable of receiving or reacting to stimuli from an outside agent, be it physical, mechanical, electrical or chemical, and this gives rise to an impulse which is conducted along the fibre. Dendrites are fibres which carry impulses to the cell body and are sometimes finely branched like a tree (see Fig. 3.1). Axons are fibres carrying impulses away from the cell body, each neurone having just one axon.

Clusters of neurone cell-bodies have a slightly grey colour and make up the *grey matter* of the nervous system. Inside the brain and spinal cord the clusters are called *nuclei*, but outside these areas they are termed *ganglia*. Nerve fibres are grouped together to form the *white matter* of the nervous system, the whiteness being due to the sheath which surrounds each fibre. White matter is found as tracts or bundles of fibres in the brain and spinal cord, as well as forming the peripheral nerves themselves.

The sheath surrounding nerve fibres acts as an insulator and protects the fibres from injury. It consists of two coats. A thick, fatty inner layer of a substance called myelin forms the *myelin sheath*. This is interrupted at intervals by gaps called *nodes of Ranvier* at which branches of the axon may leave.

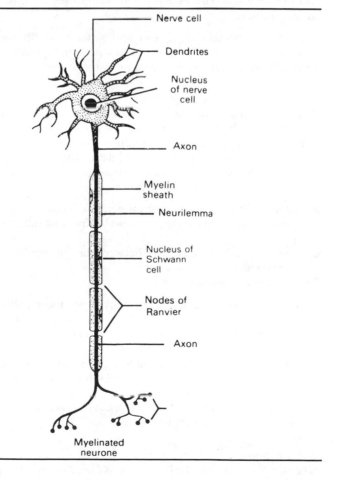

Nerve cell

Dendrites

Nucleus of nerve cell

Axon

Myelin sheath

Neurilemma

Nucleus of Schwann cell

Nodes of Ranvier

Axon

Myelinated neurone

Fig. 3.1 A neurone

A thin membrane of connective tissue, the *neurilemma*, forms the outer layer and covers the myelin sheath.

Types of nerves (briefly explained in Vol. 1, Chap. 2)

Sensory (or afferent) nerves conduct impulses to the CNS from the periphery (any part of the body outside the CNS), i.e. from sense organs to the spinal cord or brain. The sensations which are conducted to the CNS by sensory nerves include:

● common senses, originating in the skin of heat, cold or pain,
● special senses, of taste, smell, sight and hearing,
● proprioceptor senses, originating chiefly in muscles, tendons and joints often playing an important part in maintaining balance and posture.

Motor (or efferent) nerves conduct impulses away from the brain or spinal cord to or towards muscles and glands stimulating them to carry out their various functions.

Mixed nerves contain both sensory and motor nerve fibres enclosed in the same sheath of connective tissue and lie outside the spinal cord. In the spinal cord the fibres are arranged in separate *tracts* or bundles.

Transmission of nerve impulses

This involves more than one neurone, i.e. two or more neurones conduct impulses from the periphery to the spinal cord or brain and back to the periphery. The impulse begins in receptors (distal ends of sensory neurones) and ends in effectors (muscle or glandular cells). The junction where nerve impulses are transmitted from one neurone to another is called a *synapse* (see Fig. 3.2(a)). The synapse comprises:

● small swellings at the end of the terminal branch of the axon, called a *synaptic knob* (containing a chemical compound called a *neurotransmitter*;
● a *synaptic cleft*, the tiny space between the synaptic knob and a dendrite or cell body; and
● the *plasma membrane*.

As nerve fibres of connecting nerve cells do not touch each other, impulses are relayed from one to another by chemical means across the synapse between them. In most cases it requires an impulse to cross more than one synapse to cause the desired action (see Fig. 3.2(b)). Variations in transmission of impulses are mainly due to changes in the synapses. A synapse is rather like a set of traffic lights, whereby it can go green to speed up the traffic, amber to slow it down, or red to bring it to a complete halt, all dependent on outside influences. For instance, powerful pain-killers block all messages of pain by preventing impulses from crossing the synapses.

Reflex action

In certain circumstances the brain or spinal cord can react automatically to a

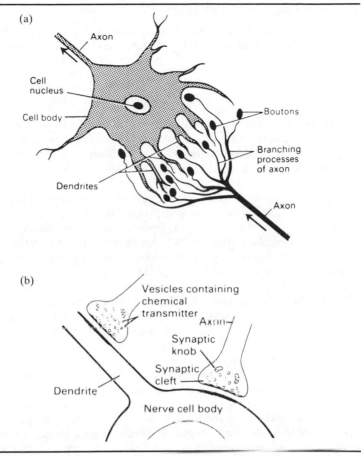

Fig. 3.2 (a) Diagram of a synapse
(b) Magnified synapse

sensory stimulus without the involvement of conscious thought. Such an action is called a reflex action. Spinal reflexes involving the spinal cord but not the brain include:

1 if the hand touches a hot object, muscles react immediately and automatically to remove the hand from the object;
2 a tap on the patella ligament produces a knee jerk;
3 tickling the sole of the foot causes the toes to bend downwards.

Reflexes occurring at the base of the brain include coughing, sneezing and vomiting. A reflex action involves the stimulus passing along a sensory nerve, being transmitted by connector neurones in the brain or spinal cord to motor nerve fibres and so to muscles. This pathway for an automatic reaction is called a reflex arc.

The central nervous system (*CNS*)

The central nervous system consists of the brain and spinal cord. These are surrounded by cerebrospinal fluid (CSF) enclosed by membranes known as *meninges*.

The brain

The brain lies within the cranial cavity of the skull and in most adults it weighs about 3 lb (1.36 kg). It is made up of billions of nerve cells intricately connected with each other. The parts of the brain are the cerebrum, the brain stem (which includes the midbrain, pons varolii and medulla oblongata), and the cerebellum (or hind brain).

The *cerebrum* is the largest and main portion of the brain and occupies the anterior and middle cranial fossae (depressions) (see Fig. 3.3). It is divided into two hemispheres which control opposite sides of the body, e.g. damage to the right hemisphere affects the left side of the body. The hemispheres are made up of a folded outer layer, or *cortex*, of grey cells several layers deep, covering a central core of white matter (nerve fibres).

The cerebral cortex is divided into functional regions and is the part of the brain most directly responsible for mental activities involving consciousness, memory, perception, thought, mental ability and intellect. It also has connections, direct or indirect, with all parts of the body as it receives information from the senses and directs the conscious movements of the body (see Fig. 3.4 showing the functional areas).

Beneath the cortex, deep within the cerebral hemispheres lies the *thalamus* where body sensations, i.e. from the skin, viscera and the special sense organs, are transmitted before distribution to the cerebrum.

Below the thalamus, at the base of the cerebrum, lies the *hypothalamus*, the head of the autonomic nervous system with separate centres for both sympathetic and parasympathetic regulations and which influences the release of hormones by the pituitary gland (see endocrine system). Therefore, it is important in controlling hunger, thirst, body temperature and the regulation of body fluids.

The *midbrain* forms the upper part of the brain stem and lies between the cerebrum above and the pons varolii below. It is composed of nerve cells and nerve fibres connecting the cerebrum with the lower parts of the brain and the spinal cord and is concerned with sight reflexes and hearing.

The *pons varolii* forms the middle part of the brain stem and lies between the midbrain and the medulla oblongata. It is composed mainly of nerve fibres which form a bridge (pons means bridge) linking the vital centre of the brain stem with the balancing control of the cerebellum (see below).

The *medulla oblongata* forms the lower portion of the brain which extends from the pons varolii above and is continuous with the spinal cord. In the medulla, the tracts of nerves, both motor and sensory, cross over, left to right and right to left, and this unaccountable fact causes the left hemisphere of the cerebrum to control the right half of the body and the right hemisphere to control the left half of the body. This part of the brain also contains the centres that are concerned with the function of the visceral organs (i.e. stomach, lungs and heart), and the respiratory system.

The *cerebellum* (or little brain or hind brain) is attached to the back of the brain stem beneath the curve of the cerebrum (see Fig. 3.3). It has an outer

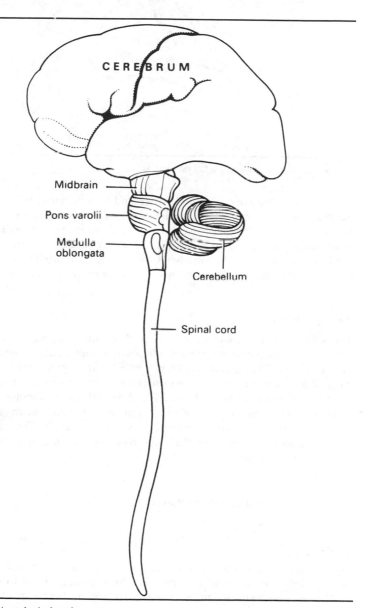

Fig. 3.3 Brain and spinal cord

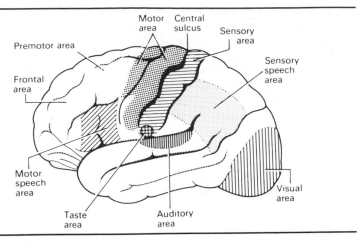

Fig. 3.4 The cerebrum showing the functional areas

grey cortex and a core of white matter and is connected, by way of the midbrain, with the motor area of the cortex and with the spinal cord. The function of the cerebellum is to maintain equilibrium and co-ordination by maintaining muscle tone and balance, i.e. as it operates entirely below the level of consciousness, the impulses from the cerebellum influence the contraction of skeletal muscle so that balance and posture are maintained.

The spinal cord

The spinal cord (approximately 18 in or 45 cm long) begins at the medulla oblongata where it emerges from the foramen magnum (large opening at the base of the skull) and ends between the first and second lumbar vertebra, where it tapers as the cauda equina and is the nervous tissue link between the brain and the rest of the body (see Fig. 3.6). The cord is composed of an inner core of grey matter in which nerve cells predominate and an outer layer of white matter in which myelinated nerve fibres prevail. The spinal cord conducts impulses to and from the brain and controls many automatic muscular activities (reflexes).

The meninges and cerebrospinal fluid

The meninges are in three layers:

1 The dura mater
(a) The *cerebral dura mater* consists of two layers of dense fibrous tissue, the outer layer lining the skull and the inner layer uniting with it to provide a protective covering for the brain except where venous sinuses are formed and where the dura mater forms partitions, i.e.

- the *falx cerebri* projects downward into the longitudinal fissure (groove or furrow) between the two cerebral hemispheres; and
- the *tentorium cerebelli* separates the cerebellum from the occipital lobe of the cerebrum.

(b) The *spinal dura mater*, similar to the cerebral dura mater, encloses the spinal cord and begins at the foramen magnum and ends at the second sacral vertebra and thereafter forms a slender filament known as the *filum terminale* to the coccyx (see Fig. 3.5).

2. The arachnoid mater
This is a delicate membrane lying between the dura mater and the pia mater (innermost layer of the meninges). Between the dura mater and this membrane is a small space called the *subdural space* and between the arachnoid and the pia mater is the *subarachnoid space* which contains cerebrospinal fluid (see Fig. 3.5).

3. The pia mater
This is a delicate connective tissue, containing many minute blood vessels, which covers the actual surface of the brain and spinal cord.
The brain and the spinal cord are also surrounded by cerebrospinal fluid (CSF). It is contained in the subarachnoid of the meninges and circulates in the four ventricles of the brain (i.e. four irregular shaped cavities) and in the central canal of the spinal cord. The CSF is secreted by the choroid plexus, which is a rich network of blood vessels derived from the pia mater in each of the brain's ventricles. It is a clear, slightly alkaline fluid and contains glucose, salts, enzymes and a few white cells. The fluid aids in the protection of the brain, spinal cord and meninges by acting as a watery cushion surrounding them to absorb any shocks. It protects the nervous tissue from harmful chemicals and also provides nutrients for the nervous system.

The peripheral nervous system (PNS)

The PNS consists of 12 pairs of cranial nerves (detailed in Vol. 1, Chap. 4, Figs. 4.10 and 4.11 and Tables 4.5–4.7) and 31 pairs of spinal nerves leaving the spinal cord (see Fig. 3.6). The spinal nerves have no special names but are numbered according to the level of the spinal column from which they emerge and these are:

- 8 cervical,
- 12 thoracic,
- 5 lumbar,
- 5 sacral,
- 1 coccygeal.

The 31 pairs of spinal nerves arise segmentally from two roots, i.e. motor nerves fibres forming an *anterior* root unite with the sensory nerve of a

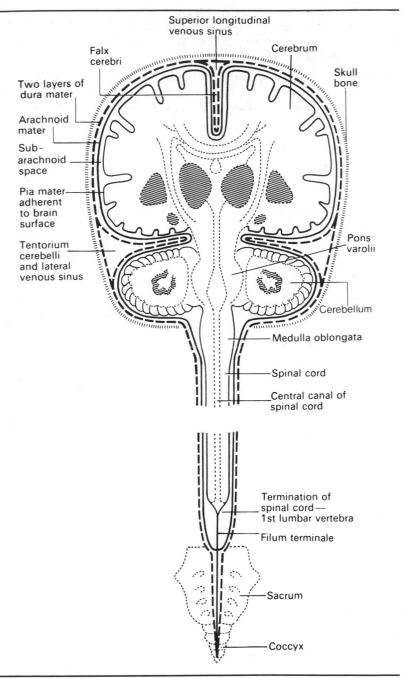

Fig. 3.5 The meninges covering brain and spinal cord

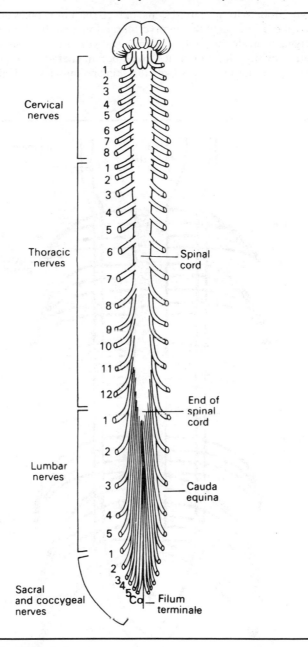

Fig. 3.6 The spinal cord and spinal nerves

posterior root to form a mixed spinal nerve. This union takes place before the nerve passes through the intervertebral foramen but immediately after emerging it divides again into anterior and posterior primary divisions. The anterior divisions form branches which become nerve *plexuses* for the limbs and the posterior divisions supply the skin and muscles of the back (see Fig. 3.7).

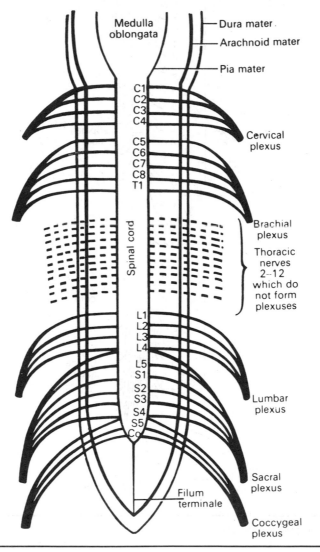

Fig. 3.7 Diagram showing the membranes covering the spinal cord, spinal nerves and the plexuses they form

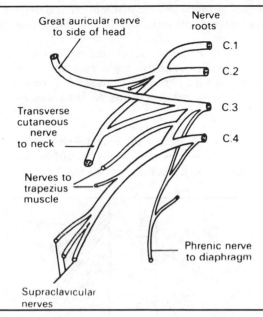

Great auricular nerve
to side of head

Nerve
roots

C.1

C.2

C.3

C.4

Transverse
cutaneous
nerve
to neck

Nerves to
trapezius
muscle

Phrenic nerve
to diaphragm

Supraclavicular
nerves

Fig. 3.8 The cervical plexus

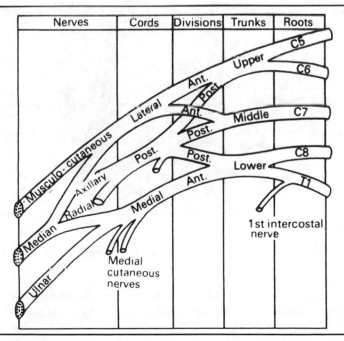

Nerves	Cords	Divisions	Trunks	Roots

Upper

C5

C6

Ant.

Post.

Lateral

Ant.

Middle

C7

Post.

Musculo-cutaneous

Post.

Post.

Lower

C8

Axillary

Ant.

T1

Radial

Medial

Median

1st intercostal
nerve

Medial
cutaneous
nerves

Ulnar

Fig. 3.9 The brachial plexus

The cervical plexus   is formed by the first four cervical nerves. The phrenic nerves which supply the diaphragm also arise from this plexus (see Fig. 3.8).

The brachial plexus   lies under the clavicle and in the axilla and is formed by the four lower cervical nerves and the first thoracic nerve (see Fig. 3.9).

It should be noted that the 12 pairs of thoracic nerves do not intermingle to form plexuses but branches run directly to intercostal muscles and the skin of the thorax.

The lumbosacral plexus   lies deep in the abdomen and provides the principal spinal nerves to the lower limbs. The lumbar plexus is formed by the first three and part of the fourth lumbar nerves (see Fig. 3.10). The sacral plexus

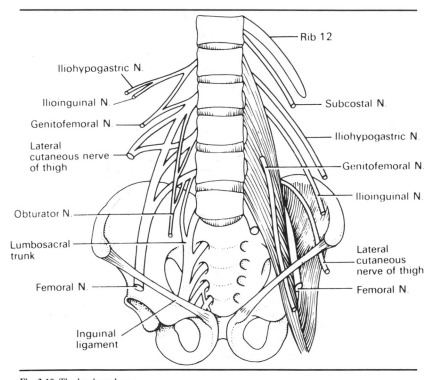

Fig. 3.10 The lumbar plexus

is formed by the first, second and third sacral nerves and by the lumbosacral trunk, formed by part of the fourth lumbar and fifth lumbar nerves.

The sacral and coccygeal plexuses   are very small plexuses formed by part of the fourth sacral nerve, fifth sacral nerve and coccygeal nerves (see Fig. 3.11).

Table 3.1 gives a summary of the main spinal nerves.

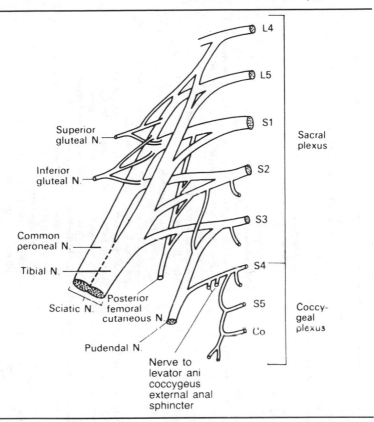

Fig. 3.11 The sacral and coccygeal plexuses

The autonomic nervous system

The autonomic nervous system is not, as the name suggests, a separate system. It is dependent on the CNS with which it is connected by afferent and efferent nerves. It is the part of the nervous system which is responsible for the control of bodily functions that are not consciously directed, i.e. regular beating of the heart, intestinal movements, glandular secretion and size of the pupils of the eyes. Generally speaking, most autonomic neurones are efferent neurones and they conduct impulses away from the brain stem or spinal cord to effector organs and tissues. The autonomic nervous system is divided into two parts, i.e. sympathetic (thoracolumbar outflow) and parasympathetic (craniosacral outflow).

Sympathetic nervous system

Ganglia (i.e. a general term to designate a group of nerve cell bodies) of this system lie on either side of the anterior surface of the spinal column. Because

Table 3.1 Spinal nerves

Spinal nerve roots		Plexus	Origin	Distribution
Cervical	C1	Cervical	Lesser occipital	Sensory nerve to back of head, front of neck and upper part of shoulder.
	C2		Great auricular	
	C3		Transverse cutaneous nerve of neck	
	C4		Anterior, middle and posterior supraclavicular	Motor nerve to numerous neck muscles i.e. sternocleidomastoid and trapezius
	C3–5	Cervical	Phrenic	Diaphragm (for respiration)
	C5	Brachial	Subscapular	Subscapular and teres major muscles
	C5–6	Brachial	Suprascapular	Supraspinous and infraspinous muscles
	C5–6	Brachial	Axillary (circumflex)	Deltoid and teres minor muscles and skin over shoulder
	C5–6–7	Brachial	Musculocutaneous	Biceps and brachialis muscles and skin of radial side of arm
	C5–6–7–8–T1	Brachial	Radial	Extensors of arm, forearm and hand
	C5–6–7–8–T1	Brachial	Median	Most flexor muscles on front of forearm and hand
	C5–6–7	Brachial	Long thoracic	Anterior serratus muscle
	C7–8	Brachial	Thoracodorsal	Latissimus dorsi muscle
	C7–8–T1	Brachial	Ulna	Flexor carpi ulnaris and part of flexor digitorum profundus, some muscles of the hand
	C8–T1	Brachial	Medial cutaneous	Sensory nerve to inner surface of arm and forearm
Lumbar	T12	Lumbosacral	Iliohypogastric	Skin over side of buttocks and over pubis
	T12–L1	Lumbosacral	Ilioinguinal	Anterior scrotal or anterior labial region
	L1–2	Lumbosacral	Genitofemoral	Skin of external genitalia and inguinal region
	L2–3	Lumbosacral	Lateral cutaneous nerve of thigh	Skin of lateral aspect and front of thigh
	L2–3–4	Lumbosacral	Femoral	Motor to quadriceps, sartorius and iliacus muscles, Sensory to front of thigh and medial side of lower leg (saphenous nerve)
	L2–3–4	Lumbosacral	Obturator	Gracilis, long and short adductor muscles, skin of medial side of thigh and leg
	L4–(5)	Lumbosacral	Lumbosacral trunk	Pelvis

	Segments	Plexus	Nerve	Distribution
Sacral	L4–S3	Lumbosacral	Sciatic (which divides at the level of the middle of the femur into:	Buttocks, descending through posterior aspect of the thigh supplying hamstring muscles
			Tibial	Leg and foot
			Sural	Main branch of the tibial nerve supplying tissues at the back of the leg and in the area of the heel, ankle and dorsum of the foot
	L5	Lumbosacral	Common peroneal (including deep peroneal (anterior tibial) and superficial peroneal (musculocutaneous))	Evertors and dorsiflexors of the foot and lateral surface of leg and dorsal surface of the foot
	L5–S2	Lumbosacral	Gluteal inferior	Gluteus maximus muscle
	L4–S1	Lumbosacral	Gluteal superior	Gluteal muscles
	S1–3	Lumbosacral	Posterior cutaneous nerve of the thigh	Skin of inferior gluteal region, posterior surface of thigh and leg; external genitalia
	S2–4	Lumbosacral	Pudendal	Muscles of the pelvic floor; skin in the area of the coccyx

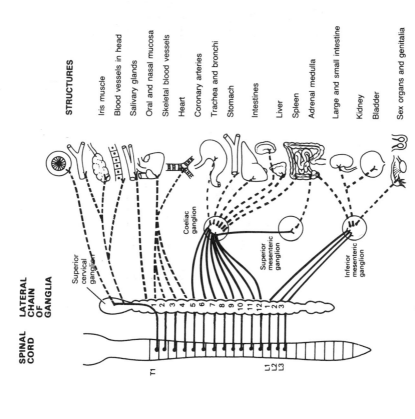

SPINAL CORD	LATERAL CHAIN OF GANGLIA	STRUCTURES	EFFECTS OF STIMULATION
	Superior cervical ganglion	Iris muscle	Pupil dilated Slightly relaxed
		Blood vessels in head	Constricted
		Salivary glands	Secretion inhibited
		Oral and nasal mucosa	Mucus secretion inhibited
		Skeletal blood vessels	Dilated
	Coeliac ganglion	Heart	Rate and force of contraction increased
		Coronary arteries	Dilated
		Trachea and bronchi	Slight vasoconstriction
		Stomach	Peristalsis reduced Sphincters closed
	Superior mesenteric ganglion	Intestines	Peristalsis and tone decreased Vasoconstriction
		Liver	Glycogen → glucose conversion increased
		Spleen	Contracted
	Inferior mesenteric ganglion	Adrenal medulla	Adrenalin and noradrenalin secretion increased
		Large and small intestine	Motility reduced Sphincters closed
		Kidney	Urine secretion decreased
		Bladder	Wall relaxed Sphincter closed
		Sex organs and genitalia	Generally blood vessels constricted

Fig. 3.12 The sympathetic outflow, the main structures supplied and the effects of stimulation.
Solid lines – preganglionic fibres, broken lines – postganglionic fibres

short fibres connect them to each other, they look like two chains of beads and are often referred to as 'sympathetic chain ganglia'. Each chain (usually made up of 22 ganglia) extends from the second cervical vertebra down to the level of the coccyx. Preganglionic fibres emerge from cell bodies in the thoracic and first three lumbar segments of the spinal cord and postganglia fibres are distributed to the heart, smooth muscle and glands of the entire body.

Other sympathetic ganglia are placed in relation to these two chains of ganglia and are situated in the abdominal cavity close to the arteries of the same names, i.e. coeliac, superior mesenteric and inferior mesenteric ganglion.

The reactions of the sympathetic nervous system are directed towards mobilisation of the resources of the body to meet danger or an emotional crisis, e.g. by increasing heart rate and breathing rate, by raising blood pressure and slowing digestive processes. This therefore prepares the body for 'flight or fight' and it also antagonises the effects of the parasympathetic nervous system.

Fig. 3.12 shows the structures supplied and the effects of stimulation.

Parasympathetic nervous system

The preganglionic fibres which emerge from cell bodies in the cranial nerves III, VII, IX and X, and the first three sacral nerves supply motor nerves to the smooth muscles of the internal organs and to cardiac muscles. The reactions of the parasympathetic nervous system are to antagonise the sympathetic nervous system, whereby it has a more restrictive effect. It is concerned with conserving and restoring energy by slowing the heart rate, lowering the blood pressure and promoting digestion. Fig. 3.13 shows the structures supplied and the effects of stimulation.

Disorders, diseases and infections of the nervous system

Disorders, diseases and infections of the nervous system are obviously the concern of the medical profession. However, there are few which the beauty therapist may recognise. For instance, *neuralgia* (which is a pain in a nerve or along the course of one or more nerves) or *neuritis* (which is the inflammation of a nerve) attack the peripheral nerves that link the brain and spinal cord with muscles, skin, etc. Liaison with the client's doctor may result in the beauty therapist's being able to help relieve pain through exercise, massage and advice for a nutritious diet containing extra vitamins, especially of the B group.

Sciatica   is not always the result of a slipped or herniated intervertebral disc. It may be the result of a back injury or arthritis of the spine or simply pressure on the nerve from certain types of exertion where massage and icepacks may relieve the pain.

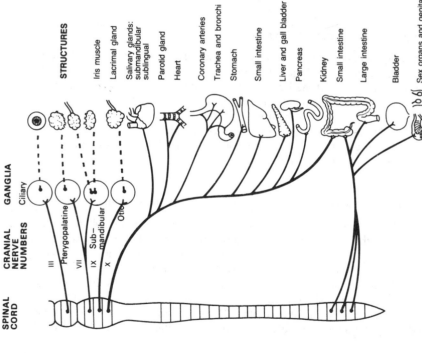

SPINAL CORD	CRANIAL NERVE NUMBERS	GANGLIA	STRUCTURES	EFFECTS OF STIMULATION
	III	Ciliary	Iris muscle	Pupil constricted / Contracted
	VII	Pterygopalatine	Lacrimal gland	Tear secretion increased
		Sub-mandibular	Salivary glands: submandibular sublingual	Saliva secretion increased
	IX	Otic	Parotid gland	Saliva secretion increased
	X		Heart	Rate and force of contraction decreased
			Coronary arteries	Constricted
			Trachea and bronchi	Constricted
			Stomach	Secretion of gastric juice and motility increased
			Small intestine	Digestion and absorption increased
			Liver and gall bladder	Blood vessels dilated / Secretion of bile increased / Secretion of pancreatic juice increased
			Pancreas	
			Kidney	Urine secretion increased
			Small intestine	Secretion of intestinal juice and motility increased
			Large intestine	Secretions and motility increased / Sphincters relaxed
			Bladder	Muscle of wall contracted / Sphincters relaxed
			Sex organs and genitalia	Male: erection / Female: variable; depending on stage in cycle

Fig. 3.13 The parasympathetic outflow, the main structures supplied and the effects of stimulation. Solid lines – peganglionic fibres, broken lines – postganglionic fibres

Herpes zosta (shingles) is also a nerve ailment, with symptoms of pain and small blisters following the path of the affected nerve. Although a client may have recovered completely it is advisable to avoid electrical (faradic) treatments on the body for six months as the electrical current stimulates the sensory nerve endings.

Epilepsy is another disorder of the nervous system that is usually controlled by medication, but there are treatments that should not be given by the beauty therapist, i.e. heat therapy (including the sun-bed) and electrical stimulation.

The more you understand of the nervous system, the greater will be the advice that you can give to the client.

Special senses

The function of all senses involves the reception of stimuli by sense organs and each sense organ is sensitive to a particular kind of stimulus, i.e.

- the taste buds of the tongue, to taste;
- the olfactory organs of the nose, to smell;
- the eyes, are sensitive to light; and
- the ears, to sound.

Taking the above special senses individually, these are as follows.

Sense of taste

This is the peculiar sensation caused by the contact of soluble substances with the tongue. The tongue itself is composed of muscles which can be divided into two groups, i.e. the *intrinsic muscles* of the tongue which perform all the delicate movements and the *extrinsic muscles* which attach the tongue to the surrounding parts and perform larger movements, i.e. form an important part of mastication and swallowing. The organs of taste are the *taste buds* which are found in the papillae of the tongue and are also contained in the mucous membrane of the palate and pharynx. They consist of small bundles of slender cells and nerve endings, some of which have hairlike branches that are packed together in groups and these form the projections called papillae at various places in the tongue. When a substance enters the mouth, its molecules enter the pores of the papillae and stimulate the taste buds. When this happens the substance has to be dissolved in liquid but if it is not liquid (i.e. food, meat etc.) when it enters the mouth, then it melts or is chewed and becomes mixed with saliva (see Fig. 3.14).

There are four basic tastes: sweet, salt, sour and bitter, and all other tastes are combinations of these. The sweet and salt taste buds are mainly at the tip

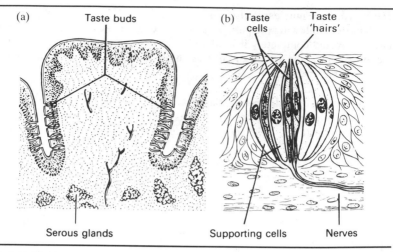

Fig. 3.14 (a) A section of the papilla. (b) A section of a taste bud – greatly magnified

of the tongue, the sour taste buds are mainly along the sides and the bitterness is tasted at the back of the tongue. The solid centre of the tongue's surface has very few taste buds. Other senses, including smell and touch, play an important role, i.e. the sense of smell may affect the appetite.

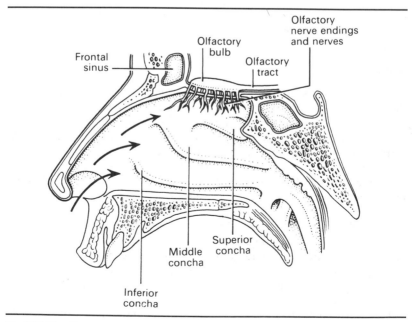

Fig. 3.15 The olfactory structures

Sense of smell

The nose has a dual function: respiration and the sense of smell. The *olfactory* or first cranial nerve supplies the end-organs of smell (see Fig. 3.15). The filaments of this nerve arise in the special cells (olfactory) in the mucous membrane of the roof of the nose above the superior nasal conchae. Nerve fibres from the cells pass through each side of the nasal septum to the olfactory bulb. From the bulb, sensation is passed along the olfactory tract by several relaying stations until it reaches the olfactory centre which lies in the temporal lobe of the cerebral hemisphere where sensation is interpreted. The

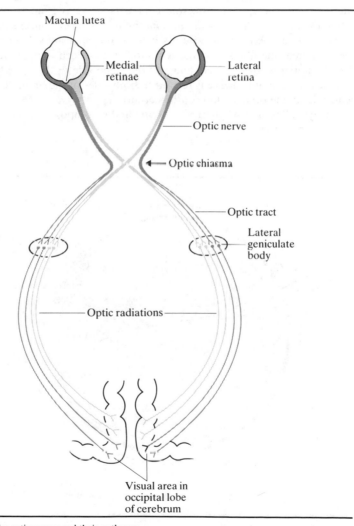

Fig. 3.16 The optic nerves and their pathways

sense of smell is very delicate and is lessened if the nasal mucous membrane becomes very dry or wet or swollen, as often happens when there is a cold in the head.

Sight and the eye

The second cranial nerve or *optic* nerve is the sensory nerve of sight and eye. The fibres of the optic nerve originate in the retina (see Fig. 3.16) and converge at the back of the eye to form the optic nerve. This runs backwards and medially, passing through the orbital cavity to enter the cranial cavity and then on to the optic chiasma where it meets the nerve from the other eye. When the fibres reach the *optic chiasma* the nerve fibres from the nasal side of each retina (medial retinae) cross over to the opposite side of the optic tract, whereas the fibres from the temporal side of each retina (lateral retinae) do not cross over but continue on the same side of the optic tract. By this means, each optic nerve is related to both sides of the brain. The visual centre lies in the occipital lobe of the cerebrum.

The eyeball is almost spherical in shape and is composed of the following three layers of tissue.

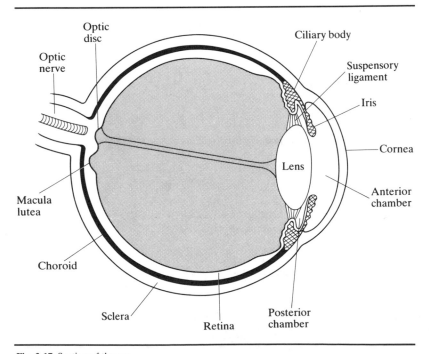

Fig. 3.17 Section of the eye

The sclera and cornea which form the outer fibrous layer. The *sclera* is the tough fibrous coat forming the white of the eye and is continuous anteriorly with the transparent window membrane, the *cornea*. This firm fibrous membrane maintains the shape of the eyeball, protects its delicate structures and gives attachment to six muscles which move the eye (see Table 3.2).

The choroid, ciliary body and iris make up the middle vascular layer. The *choroid* contains the blood vessels and is continuous in front with the *iris* which contains both circular and radial muscles controlling the central opening or pupil of the eye. The colour of the iris is determined by the number of pigment cells present. Behind the iris this layer is thickened to form the *ciliary body* containing muscle fibres which control the curvature of the lens.

The retina is the inner nervous tissue layer and this is composed of several layers of nerve cells, nerve fibres, rods and cones (see Fig. 3.17).

Summary of the function of the eye

- The cornea acts as a transparent window, allowing light to enter the eye.
- The iris acts as a curtain to protect the retina and to control the amount of light entering the eye.
- The lens, a bi-convex transparent body lying immediately behind the pupil, bends light rays reflected by objects in front of the eye, so focusing light on the retina. It is attached to the ciliary bodies of the choroid by suspensory ligaments.
- The pigmented choroid coat darkens the inner chamber of the eye and so prevents internal reflection of light inside the eye ball.
- The retina. Because the eye must function under many different circumstances, there are two different sets of nerve cells, i.e. cone- and rod-shaped. The cone-shaped cells are sensitive in bright light and the rod-shaped cells are sensitive in dim light. The cones are responsible for colour vision and a lack of or defects in a set of colour cells causes colour blindness. The optic nerve which transmits the nerve impulses from the retina to the visual centre of the brain, contains nerve fibres from the many nerve endings in the retina. The small spot where it leaves the retina does not have any light-sensitive cells and is called the blind spot or optic disc (see Fig. 3.17). The point on the retina immediately opposite the centre of the cornea is the yellow spot or macula lutea. For the clearest and most detailed vision, light must be focused on this spot.

Appendages of the eyes

Appendages of the eyes include eyebrows, eyelids, eyelashes and lacrimal apparatus.

Eyebrows are the two arches of thick skin attached to muscles beneath and covering the supraorbital margins of the frontal bone. Hairs grow obliquely from the surface of the skin and these protect the eyeball from sweat and foreign bodies.

Table 3.2 Muscles of the eye

	Location	Function
Extrinsic muscles (Voluntary)		
Superior rectus		
Inferior rectus		
Lateral rectus	All attached to the eyeball	Eye movements
Medial rectus		
Superior oblique		
Inferior oblique		
Intrinsic muscles (Involuntary)		
Iris	Iris	Iris regulates size of pupil and so controls the amount of light entering the eye
Ciliary muscle	Ciliary body	Ciliary muscle controls shape of lens

Eyelids are two tarsal plates, which are thin sheets of dense connective tissue, covered by skin and lined with conjunctiva. The latter is a delicate membrane lining the eyelids and covering the eyeball. The upper eyelid, which is larger than the lower lid, is raised by the levator palpebrae muscle and the lids are closed by the circular muscle, the orbicularis oculi (see Fig. 3.18). Along the edges of the eyelids there are modified sebaceous glands called Meibomian glands or tarsal glands which secrete an oily material. The secretion of the glands spreads over the margin of the eyelid and tends to prevent the tears from overflowing on to the cheek and it also delays the evaporation of tears.

Eyelashes are hairs attached to the free margins of the lids and they protect the eyes from dust and light.

Lacrimal apparatus is a group of organs concerned with the production and drainage of tears. The lacrimal gland, which secretes the tears is situated at the upper outer corner of the orbital cavity and its excretory ducts branch downward towards the eyeball. Tears wash down over the front of the eye and are drained from the inner angle of the eye into lacrimal ducts and then through the lacrimal sac into the naso-lacrimal duct and finally down the nose (see Fig. 3.19).

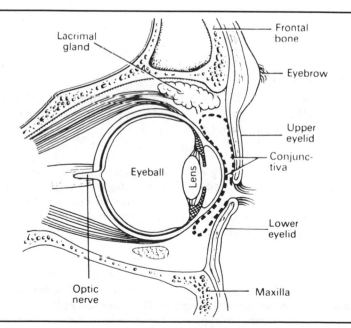

Fig. 3.18 Section of the eye and its accessory structures

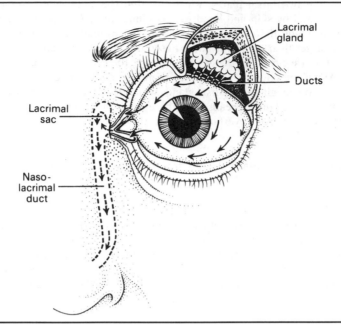

Fig. 3.19 The lacrimal apparatus. Arrow shows the direction of flow of tears

Hearing and the ear

The organ of hearing is the ear, which is divided into three sections, the external, middle, and inner ear. The nerve supplying this special sense is the eighth cranial or *auditory nerve*.

The external ear
This consists of the *auricle* (or pinna), i.e. the part projecting from the side of the head which has a *lobule* (the soft part at the lower extremity) and the *helix* which is the most prominent outer part which is ridged and grooved (see Fig. 3.20). There is a small canal about 1 in (2.5 cm) long called the *external acoustic meatus* which leads from the pinna and conveys the vibrations of sound to the *tympanic membrane* or eardrum.

The middle ear
This is also called the *tympanic cavity*. It is a very small chamber containing air and three ossicles (or small bones). These are the malleus (hammer), incus (anvil) and stapes (stirrup) and are all held in position by fine ligaments.

The malleus is attached to the tympanic membrane and the stapes connects with the oval window (fenestra ovalis), an area of fibrous tissue in the wall of the inner ear. This chain of bones serves to transmit the vibrations of sound from the ear drum to the inner ear. Then the middle ear opens into the eustachian tube which is a bony and cartilaginous tube that connects the tympanic cavity with the nasal part of the pharynx and equalises pressure on either side of the eardrum.

This equalisation of pressure against the inner and outer surfaces of the tympanic membrane prevents membrane rupture or discomfort that varying pressures produce. For instance, descending in an aeroplane often causes discomfort but by chewing, increased swallowing or yawning, air spreads rapidly through the open tube and this relieves the discomfort in the ears.

The inner ear

The inner ear is situated within the temporal bone of the cranium where it forms a complicated cavity known as the *bony labyrinth* containing a fluid called *perilymph*. The bony labyrinth consists of three parts:

1 *the vestibule* is a small cavity behind the oval window and leads to the other two parts;
2 three *semicircular canals* in different planes lead out and back to the vestibule and are concerned with balance and awareness of the position of the head;
3 the *cochlea* is a spiral tube resembling a snail shell and contains the nerve endings of the auditory nerve.

A *membranous labyrinth* floats in the perilymph and follows the shape of the bony labyrinth. It is itself hollow and contains a fluid called *endolymph*. The membranous cochlea encloses the cochlear duct which in addition to endolymph also contains the *organ of Corti* from which sensory nerve fibres for

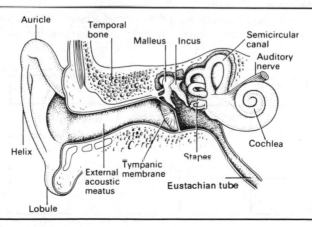

Fig. 3.20 The parts of the ear

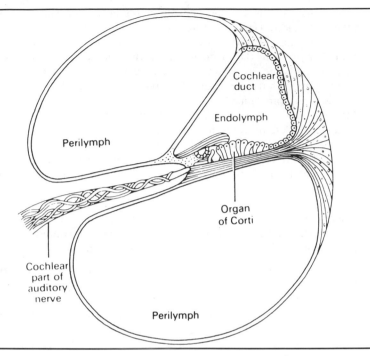

Fig. 3.21 A section of the membranous cochlea showing the organ of Corti

hearing arise. These form the cochlear nerve, a branch of the eighth cranial nerve or auditory nerve which transmits the stimulus to the centre of hearing in the brain. A second branch of the auditory nerve goes to the membranous semicircular canals for the sense of position (see Fig. 3.21).

The mechanism of hearing
Sound waves in the air pass through the external acoustic meatus causing the tympanic membranes to vibrate. These vibrations move the malleus and

EXTERNAL EAR	MIDDLE EAR	INNER EAR		
Sound waves in air	Mechanical movement of ossicles	Perilymph Fluid wave	Endolymph Fluid wave → Organ of Corti	Fluid wave
→ _Tympanic membrane_	→ _Oval window_	→ _Cochlear membrane_		→ _Round window_

Fig. 3.22 Summary of the transmission of sound through ear

when the malleus vibrates, it moves the incus, which moves the stapes against the oval window. At this point fluid conduction of sound waves through the perilymph begins. Since fluid is incompressible the perilymph can only vibrate if a second fibrous window (the round window or fenestra rotunda), also in the wall of the inner ear, bulges outwards as the oval window is pressed inwards. Vibrations of the perilymph are transmitted through the membrane to the endolymph in the cochlea duct where the stimuli reaches the nerve endings in the organ of Corti, to be transmitted to the brain by the auditory nerve (see Fig. 3.22).

The endocrine system

The endocrine system and the nervous system both function to achieve and maintain homeostasis or stability of our internal environment. The endocrine system consists of organs or ductless glands, so named because the secretions they make, i.e. *hormones*, do not leave the glands by means of a duct but pass directly from the cells into the bloodstream. Hormones act as chemical messengers to body organs (target organs) or tissue, stimulating certain life processes and retarding others. Growth, reproduction, sexual attributes and even mental conditions and personality traits are dependent on hormones (see Fig. 3.23).

The endocrine system consists of the following glands.

The pituitary gland

The pituitary gland, although only the size of a pea, has been described as 'the master gland of the body' and, together with the hypothalamus, it controls the activity of many other endocrine glands. It lies at the base of the skull, in the hypophyseal fossa of the sphenoid bone below the hypothalamus, to which it is attached by a stalk. It consists of the anterior and posterior lobes.

The anterior lobe (adenohypophysis) is an upgrowth from the pharynx and is glandular in nature. It secretes many hormones including the growth hormone (or *somatotrophic* hormone) which controls the bones and muscles and in this way determines the overall size of the individual. It produces *thyrotrophic* hormones which regulate the thyroid, *adrenocorticotrophic* hormones which regulate the adrenal cortex, *gonadotrophic* hormones for both male and female gonad activity, and also *metabolic* hormones.

The posterior lobe (neurohypophysis) is derived from a downgrowth from the base of the brain which is in close proximity to the pituitary gland. It produces two hormones:

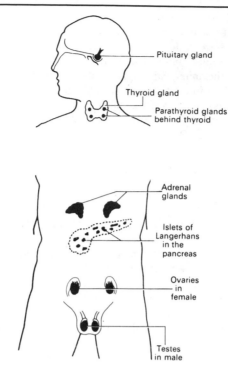

Fig. 3.23 Diagram of the positions in the body of the endocrine glands

- *oxytocin* which causes the uterine muscles to contract and also causes the mammary glands to contract during breast-feeding;
- *vasopressin* is an antidiuretic hormone (ADH).

Signals transmitted from the hypothalamus control almost all the secretions by the pituitary gland (see Fig. 3.24 and Table 3.3).

The thyroid gland

The thyroid gland is situated in the lower part of the front of the neck with two lateral lobes lying on either side of the trachea, joined in front by a narrow isthmus. It secretes *thyroxine* and *triiodothyronine*. Thyroxine controls the general metabolism but both hormones contain iodine (see Fig. 3.25 and Table 3.3).

The parathyroid glands

There are two pairs of parathyroid glands located on the dorsal part of the thyroid gland and their secretion regulates the blood calcium and phosphorus levels (see Fig. 3.26 and Table 3.3).

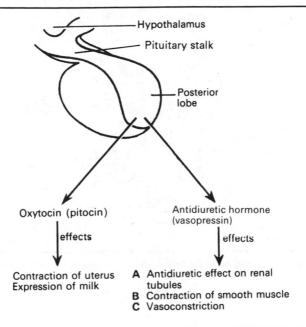

Fig. 3.24 The parts of the pituitary gland and its relation to the hypothalamus

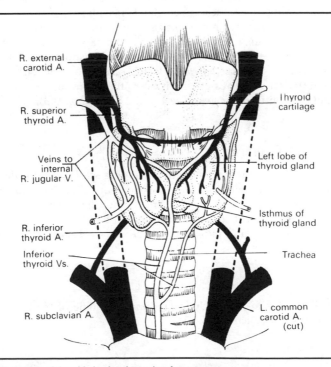

Fig. 3.25 Position of thyroid gland and associated structures

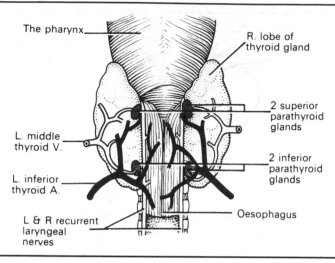

The pharynx

R. lobe of thyroid gland

2 superior parathyroid glands

L. middle thyroid V.

2 inferior parathyroid glands

L. inferior thyroid A.

Oesophagus

L & R recurrent laryngeal nerves

Fig. 3.26 The positions of the parathyroid glands and their related structures viewed from behind

The adrenal (suprarenal) glands

There are two small adrenal glands situated one on top of each kidney enclosed within the renal fascia. Each gland is composed of two parts. The outer part is the *cortex* which produces a number of hormones called corticoids and their function is to control sodium and potassium balance, increase the storage of glucose and effect the production of sex hormones. The inner part, the *medulla*, produces *adrenalin* which raises blood pressure by constriction of smaller blood vessels and it raises the blood sugar by increasing the output of sugar from the liver (see Fig. 3.27 and Table 3.3).

The islets of Langerhans

The islets of Langerhans are small groups of cells scattered throughout the pancreas which secrete glucagon and from the more abundant *beta cell*, the hormone *insulin*. The secretions pass directly into the pancreatic veins and circulate throughout the body. Insulin regulates the sugar level in the blood and the conversion of sugar into heat and energy (see Table 3.3).

The pineal gland (or body)

The pineal gland is a small body located in the middle of the brain which secretes a hormone called *melatonin*.

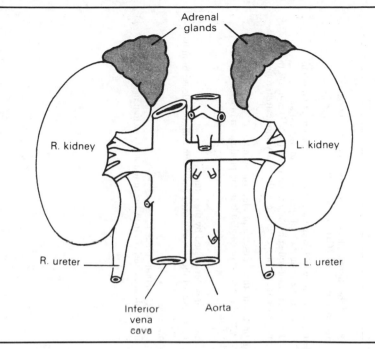

Fig. 3.27 The positions of the adrenal glands and some of their associated structures

The gonads

The gonads or sex glands, consist of the *testes* in the male and the *ovaries* in the female. Besides producing sperm and ova, respectively, they manufacture hormones responsible for the special characteristics of the male and female (see Table 3.3).

Some disorders of various glands

Hypersecretion (excessive) and hyposecretion (diminished) of hormones can cause an imbalance both in mind and body. The following disorders may help the therapist to understand a client's medical history.

Disorders of the pituitary gland

These include prolonged hypersecretion of the growth hormone which results in excessive growth of bones, enlargement of internal organs, a rise in blood pressure and reduced glucose tolerance. If this occurs before ossification of bones is complete, i.e. in childhood, then the child becomes an unusually tall adult. If the abnormality is extreme it is termed *gigantism*. However, if this

Table 3.3 Brief summary of the function of endocrine glands

Glands	Hormone secreted	Action of hormone
Pituitary		
Anterior lobe	Thyrotrophic hormone (TSH)	Controls the activity of the thyroid gland in the production of thyroxin
	Somatotrophic (GH)	Stimulates the growth of the body (Growth hormone)
	Gonadotrophic hormones i.e. (FSH)	Follicle-stimulating hormone which stimulates the development of Graafian follicles in the ovary and the formation of spermatoza in the testis
	(LH) & (ICSH)	Luteinising (LH) or interstitial-cell-stimulation hormone (ICSH) controls the secretion of the oestrogens and progesterone in the ovary and testosterone in the testis
	Prolactin	After childbirth prolactin stimulates the production of milk
	Adrenocorticotrophic hormone (ACTH)	Controls the activity of the suprarenal glands in the production of cortisol from the cortex of the gland
Posterior lobe	Antidiuretic hormone (ADH) Vasopressin	Regulates the amount of water passed by the kidneys
	Oxytocin	Stimulates the contraction of the uterus during childbirth and the release of milk during breast feeding
Thyroid	Thyroxine	Controls metabolic rate
	Triiodothyronine	Stimulates metabolism (catabolic phase)
Parathyroid	Parathormone (PTH)	Regulates calcium metabolism and controls the amount of calcium in blood and bone

Gland	Hormone	Function
Adrenal Cortex	3 groups: Glucocorticoids, i.e. Cortisol (hydrocortisone) Corticosterone	Tend to increase amount of sugar in blood and are concerned with metabolism, growth, renal function and muscle tone
	Mineralocorticoids Aldosterone	Increases the reabsorption of sodium and water and the excretion of potassium by the kidneys
	All corticoids are important for defence against stress or injury to tissues	
	Androgens	Govern certain secondary sex characteristics
Medulla	Adrenaline (epinephrine)	Converts glycogen to glucose when needed by muscles for energy, increases heart beat rate and dilates bronchioles
	Noradrenaline (norepinephrine)	Raises the blood pressure by stimulating the muscle fibres in the walls of the blood vessels causing them to contract
Islets of Langerhans	Insulin	Promotes metabolism of carbohydrates i.e. stimulates the uptake of glucose, amino acids and fats
	Glucagon	Increases blood glucose concentration
Ovaries	Oestrogen	Secreted by the ovary, promotes development and maintenance of female secondary sex characteristics
	Progesterone	Secreted by corpus luteum prepares uterus for implantation of fertilised ovum and effects the repair of endometrium after menstruation
Testes	Testosterone	Influences the development of the body to sexual maturity. Essential for normal functioning of male reproductive organs

overproduction occurs in the adult, there is an abnormal enlargement of hands and feet and coarse facial features and is known as *acromegaly*. The opposite condition, hyposecretion of the growth hormone before puberty, leads to *dwarfism*. It will be appreciated that these disorders are rarely seen.

Disorders of the thyroid gland

These may originate in the hypothalamus, anterior pituitary or thyroid gland but disorders can arise due to an insufficient intake of iodine in the diet. The principal effects are caused by abnormally high or low metabolic rate. A diffuse and painless enlargement of the thyroid gland is called a *simple goitre* where the gland enlarges in an attempt to compensate for the lack of iodine in the diet necessary for synthesis of thyroid hormone.

Hypersecretion of the thyroid hormone produces the disease *exophthalmic goitre* (Graves' disease) where there is increased metabolism, loss of weight, nervous irritability, muscle wasting and weakness and exophthalmos (protrusion of the eyeballs).

Hyposecretion during the formative years causes *cretinism*, a condition characterised by low metabolic rate, retarded mental and physical development. Later in life, deficient thyroid secretion produces the disease *myxoedema*. The low metabolic rate that characterises myxoedema leads to mental and physical processes becoming slower, a gain in weight, loss of hair and a thickening of the skin.

Disorders of the parathyroid glands

These include hyperparathyroidism, i.e. an excess secretion of parathormone (PTH) which causes *hypercalcemia*, or a higher than normal blood concentration of calcium. The calcium is attracted out of the bones into the blood serum and sometimes causes a bone disease or the calcium may be deposited in the kidney, causing renal stones or kidney failure.

Hypoparathyroidism is a PTH deficiency and causes *hypocalcemia*, which is a lower than normal blood concentration of calcium. This low blood calcium causes the development of cataracts (opacity of the lens) and increases neuromuscular irritability and, rarely, it produces muscle spasms and convulsions, a condition called tetany.

Disorders of the adrenal glands

These include the hypersecretion of glucocorticoids. It will be seen from Table 3.3 that these hormones relate to the adrenal cortex. Glucocorticoids tend to accelerate both the mobilisation of fats from adipose cells and the catabolism of fats by almost all kinds of cells and cause cells to transfer for their energy supply from their usual carbohydrate catabolism to fat catabolism. Therefore, excess hypersecretion can result in *Cushing's syndrome*, the symptoms of which include painful fatty swellings on the body, i.e. 'the buffalo hump' and moonlike fullness of the face and distension of the abdomen. There may also be an impairment of sexual function, high blood pressure, general weakness and sometimes an unusual growth of body hair (hirsutism).

Hyposecretion means an inadequate secretion of the cortisol hormone and in rare cases causes *Addison's disease* which results in lowering of the blood pressure, muscle weakness and wasting, darkening of the pigmentation of the skin, gastrointestinal disturbances, i.e. vomiting, diarrhoea, anorexia, and in women, loss of body hair and menstrual disturbances.

Hypersecretion of mineralocorticoids (also relating to the adrenal cortex) means an excess of aldosterone (principal mineralocorticoid) which affects kidney function causing excessive reabsorption of sodium, chloride and water and excessive excretion of potassium. Thus, a deficiency, i.e. hyposecretion of the mineralocorticoids, results in excessive loss of sodium in the urine and the retention of potassium in the extracellular fluid.

Disorders of the islets of Langerhans

Are due to either a deficiency of the hormone insulin causing *hyperglycaemia* or overproduction of insulin causing *hypoglycaemia*. Hyperglycaemia means an excess of glucose in the blood which results in loss of weight, fatigue and polyuria (excessive excretion of urine) with its accompanying thirst, hunger, dry skin, mouth and tongue. These are the common symptoms of *diabetes mellitus*. Because of poor circulation, a relatively high blood sugar level and decreased ability to repair damaged tissue, a client who is a diabetic may suffer serious complications from seemingly minor infections. Therefore, it is important to understand the contra-indications when performing treatments on a client who is a diabetic.

Hypoglycaemia means an abnormally low level of sugar (glucose) in the blood. Overproduction of insulin from the islets of Langerhans can lead to increased utilisation of glucose, so that glucose is removed from the blood at an accelerated rate. This may be tolerated by normal persons for brief periods of time without symptoms but if the blood sugar level remains very low for a prolonged period of time, symptoms such as mental confusion or hallucinations may arise as the nervous system is deprived of the glucose needed for its normal metabolic activities. This condition is often alleviated by the client's taking sugar, sweetened fruit juice or honey.

Chapter 4

Circulation of blood and lymph

The circulatory (or vascular) system is divided into two main parts:

- The blood circulatory system, consisting of the *heart*, which acts as a pump maintaining circulation throughout the body, *arteries* carrying the blood *from* the heart, *veins* carrying blood *to* the heart and *capillaries* uniting the arteries and veins (the composition of blood has been described in Vol. 1, Chap. 3, pp. 29–31 with Figs 3.7 and 3.8); and
- the lymphatic system, consisting of *lymph, lymphatic capillaries* and *vessels, ducts, nodes and organs.*

Blood circulatory system

The heart

The heart is a hollow muscular organ which serves as a pump controlling the blood flow. It is approximately 4 in (or 10 cm) in length and roughly the size of the owner's fist, and weighs about 8–9 oz (225–255 gm). The heart rests in the thorax, between the lungs and behind the sternum and lies a little more to the left than to the right (see Fig. 4.1 for the position of the heart). The walls of the heart are composed of three layers of tissue, i.e. pericardium, myocardium and endocardium. The outer covering is the *pericardium* of which there are two layers, i.e. the *visceral pericardium*, a serous membrane which is adherent to the heart and the *parietal pericardium* which is a fibrous layer. Between these two layers there is a serous fluid which, by a lubricating action, allows the heart to move freely. The *myocardium* is a muscular coat of cardiac muscle, contraction of which causes the circulation of blood and the *endocardium* is the inner lining. Internally, the heart is divided by a septum (see Fig. 4.2) and each side is further divided into two chambers by an *atrioventricular* valve into an upper chamber called the *atrium*, and a lower chamber, called the *ventricle* (see Fig. 4.3). Between the right atrium and right ventrical is the right atrioventricular valve known as the *tricuspid* valve as it has three flaps or *cusps*. Similarly, the left atrium and left ventricle are connected by the left atrioventricular valve called the *mitral* valve which has two cusps (see Fig. 4.2).

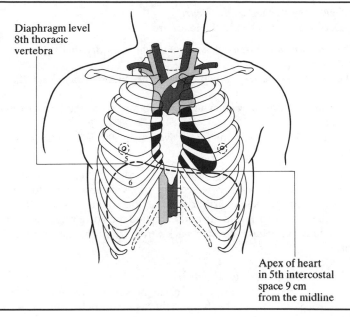

Diaphragm level
8th thoracic
vertebra

5

6

Apex of heart
in 5th intercostal
space 9 cm
from the midline

Fig. 4.1 Position of the heart in the thorax

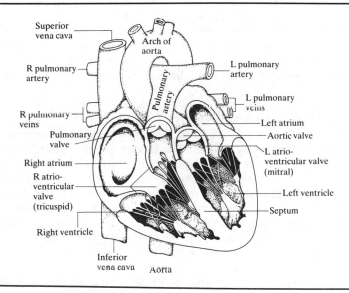

Superior
vena cava

Arch of
aorta

R pulmonary
artery

L pulmonary
artery

Pulmonary
artery

R pulmonary
veins

L pulmonary
veins

Pulmonary
valve

Left atrium

Aortic valve

Right atrium

L atrio-
ventricular valve
(mitral)

R atrio-
ventricular
valve
(tricuspid)

Left ventricle

Septum

Right ventricle

Inferior
vena cava

Aorta

Fig. 4.2 Interior of the heart

Blood vessels attached to the heart

The blood vessels attached to the heart are:

● the *superior and inferior venae cavae* which empty their blood into the right atrium;
● the *pulmonary artery* which carries the blood away from the right ventricle;
● the four *pulmonary veins* which bring blood from the lungs to the left atrium; and
● the *aorta* which carries the blood away from the left ventricle (see Fig. 4.3).

The opening of the pulmonary artery is guarded by the pulmonary valve (formed by three semilunar cusps, see Fig. 4.2) which prevents blood flowing backwards from the pulmonary artery into the right ventricle. The valve between the left ventricle and the aorta is called the aorta valve (see Fig. 4.2) and this prevents blood flowing backwards from the aorta to the left ventricle.

The flow of blood through the heart

Deoxygenated blood from the venae cavae passes into the thin-walled right atrium, through the tricuspid valve into the right ventricle (which has a fairly thick muscular wall). The right ventricle contracts and pumps blood (via the pulmonary valve) to the pulmonary artery and so to the lungs. After oxygenation in the lungs, blood passes along the four pulmonary veins into the left atrium, through the mitral valve into the left ventricle. From the left ventricle, which has a thick muscular wall, blood is then pumped through the aortic valve into the aorta and then to all parts of the body (see Fig. 4.3).

Therefore, in summary, the right side of the heart is concerned with deoxygenated blood; the left side of the heart is concerned with oxygenated blood.

Blood and nerve supply to the heart

Arterial blood is supplied to heart muscle itself by branches of the aorta, i.e. the right and left coronary arteries. The venous return is by the coronary sinus which empties into the right atrium and there are also some small channels which open into the chambers of the heart. The action of the heart is rhythmic, although its rate of contraction can be affected by impulses reaching it from the vagus and sympathetic nerves. Control by the vagus nerve (parasympathetic system) causes the heartbeat to be slowed, whereas control from the sympathetic system accelerates the rate of the heartbeat. Normally, the heart is controlled equally by the parasympathetic and sympathetic nerves but when the rate of the heartbeat is increased to meet the needs of the body in times of stress or physical exercise, the sympathetic system is stimulated.

Blood pressure

This term usually refers to the pressure of blood within the arteries and is determined by several factors, i.e. pumping action of the heart, the elasticity

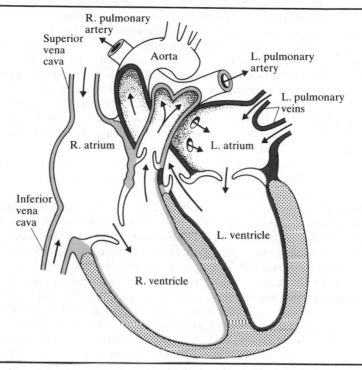

Fig. 4.3 Diagram of the flow of blood through heart

of the walls of the main arteries, the quantity of blood within the blood vessels and the blood's viscosity (thickness). The maximum pressure of each heartbeat, or *systole* is measured when the heart is pushing the blood out into the body and lungs via the pulmonary artery and the aorta, and is known as the *systolic blood pressure*. The minimum pressure is taken when the heart has filled with blood from the head, arms, lungs and body and is known as the *diastolic blood pressure*.

It is these two pressures which are measured in order to determine a client's level of blood pressure. This is usually measured in the artery of the upper arm, with a sphygmomanometer. Very simple machines can be purchased now (without the use of a stethoscope) which are useful for the beauty therapist. They have an arm cuff which should be wrapped around the client's arm with the small blood pressure meter inside placed over the artery and the bottom edge of the cuff about 1 in (2–3 cm) above the elbow joint.

The cuff is held in place with a Velcro fastener, and it is important that it is not attached too tightly; it should be loose enough to insert one or two fingers between the arm and cuff. Air is pumped into the cuff by squeezing the rubber bulb and as pressure increases, the flow of blood through the artery is momentarily checked, causing the gauge's needle on the display panel to move. A bleeping sound will be heard when the cuff pressure exceeds 160, 200, 240 and 280 mm Hg (i.e. millimetres of mercury). Keep the arm still once the cuff has been pumped up as any movement of the air tubes, the arm cuff or the blood pressure meter may lead to inaccurate results.

The compression of the arm cuff diminishes slowly, and so does the pressure on the artery. The diminishing pressure can be seen usually as small 'heart' symbol on the display panel and as soon as the blood begins to flow again the symbol will start blinking in a rhythm which corresponds with the heartbeat. This will eventually stop and the figure which appears on the left-hand side of the display panel will give the systolic pressure and the figure on the right-hand side will give the diastolic pressure. There are many manufacturers and varying designs of blood-pressure machines and it is necessary to ensure that the relevant instruction leaflet is obtained.

The use of these machines is recommended, as a precautionary measure, to the beauty therapist working in an area where heat treatments are given (i.e. saunas or steam cabinets).

Normal blood pressure can vary between the sexes, among different age groups and even between two persons of the same age and sex. It can also vary according to the time of day and the kind of activity undertaken by the client, i.e. strenuous physical activity can increase the systolic blood pressure 60–80 mm. above the normal. It also increases with age and is usually higher in women than in men. High blood pressure (hypertension) can also be influenced by diet and stress. Low blood pressure (hypotension) is rarely a cause for concern but can often happen when a client is very tired. Normally, low blood pressure is associated with long life and old age free of illness.

For young and middle-aged clients a systolic pressure of 120 and a diastolic pressure of 80, written as 120/80, is considered normal, whereas 160/95 would be considered high. However in older clients (60 years of age and over) 140–170 systolic and 80–90 diastolic would be acceptable.

During a figure consultation you may find the client is taking medication, i.e. diuretics (known as 'water tablets') or 'beta-blockers'. It is worth finding out more about the client's health as these drugs are usually prescribed to treat high blood pressure, and the latter will obviously dictate contra-indications to general heat therapy. Beauty therapists can help clients with hypertension is a small way with advice i.e.

● by keeping the weight down, as overweight clients make a lot of extra work for their circulatory system; often blood pressure will fall when excess weight is shed;
● advise regular exercise, yoga and brisk walking is excellent;
● advise clients who smoke (cigarettes or cigars) to give it up completely as the nicotine in cigarettes is rapidly absorbed into the blood stream and is known to increase blood pressure.

The pulse

The pulse is said to be the beat of the heart as felt through the walls of the arteries but what is actually felt is not the blood pulsing through the arteries, but a shock wave that travels along the fibres of the arteries as the heart contracts. The pulse can be felt wherever an artery lies near the surface and over a bone or other firm background, i.e.

radial artery   – at the wrist;
temporal artery   – at the temple;
carotid artery   – at the side of the neck;
brachial artery   – at the elbow;
femoral artery   – at the anterior side of the hip bone;
popliteal artery   – at the back of the knee; and
dorsalis pedis artery – at the instep.

However, the pulse is usually felt just inside the wrist below the thumb by placing, lightly, two or three fingers on the radial artery. In taking a pulse, the rate, rhythm and strength of the pulse are noted. The average resting rate in an adult is between 60 and 80 beats per minute although this can be affected by the following.

Exercise Walking, running, jogging or playing games will increase the rate of the pulse. When a beauty therapist is taking an exercise class, it is useful to let the clients take their own pulse rate before the exercise, immediately afterwards to check on the amount of increase in pulse rate, and finally, to check how long it takes the pulse to be restored to its resting rate. Always take into consideration the sex, as the pulse rate tends to be more rapid in females than in males, and age of the client.

Emotion The pulse rate is increased when strong emotional feelings are experienced, i.e. grief, fear, anger or excitement.

Circulation of the blood

There are in reality two independent circulatory systems within the body, each with its own pump inside the sheath of the heart.

The pulmonary circulation
This is the circulation of blood to and from the lungs, whereby the blood from the right ventricle flows through the right and left pulmonary arteries to the right and left lung. In the lungs the branches subdivide and emerge as capillaries and carbon dioxide is released in exchange for a fresh supply of oxygen. The capillaries containing oxygenated blood unite and eventually form the two pulmonary veins, i.e. one from each lung returning oxygenated blood to the left atrium of the heart.

The systemic or general circulation
In this system blood flows from the left ventricle through the aorta, carrying oxygen and nutrient material to all systems and organs of the body, and returning through the superior and inferior venae cavae to the right atrium. Figure 4.4 shows the relationship between the pulmonary and systemic

circulation. The main arteries are only major pipelines distributing blood from the heart to the various organs and in each organ, its main artery resembles a tree trunk in that it gives off numerous branches that continue to branch and re-branch. The aorta is the largest artery in the body and begins at the upper part of the left ventricle. It ascends for a short distance and then arches backwards and to the left, descending behind the heart, through the thoracic and abdominal cavities, and then divides into the right and left common iliac arteries (see Fig. 4.5 and Table 4.1(b)).

The aorta and main arteries of the limbs are shown on Fig. 4.6 and Tables 4.1(a), (b) and (c) give their origin and principal branches.

It may be easier to learn the names of the blood vessels and the relation of the vessels to each other from diagrams than from descriptions. Many of the main arteries have corresponding veins bearing the same name and located alongside or near the arteries. Figure 4.7 shows the venae cavae and the main veins of the limbs and Table 4.2(a) and (b) give their regions. Venous blood from the head, neck, upper limbs and thoracic cavity (with the exception of the lungs) drains into the superior vena cava, whereas the blood from the

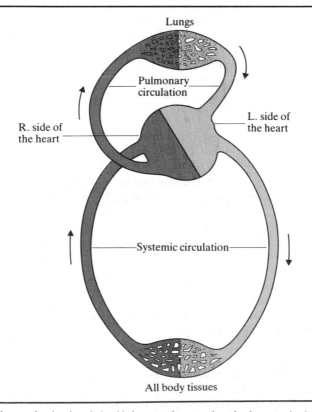

Fig. 4.4 Diagram showing the relationship between the systemic and pulmonary circulation

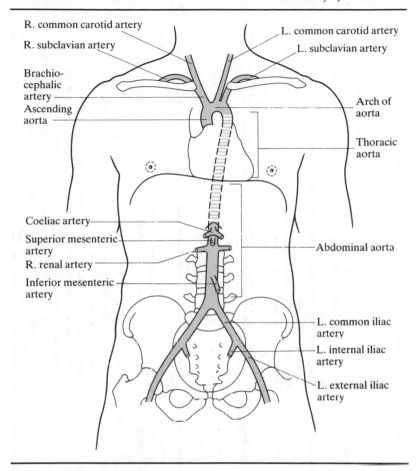

Fig. 4.5 Aorta and its main branches

lower limbs and abdomen (i.e. paired testicular, ovarian, renal and adrenal veins) drains into the inferior vena cava.

So far, the circulatory system has been discussed where venous blood passes from the tissues to the heart in a simple direct route. However, blood from certain organs in the abdominal cavity passes through the liver before entering the inferior vena cava via the *portal circulation*. Veins from the spleen, stomach, pancreas, gall-bladder and intestines send their blood to the liver by means of the *portal vein*. As will be seen by Figure 4.8 this vein is formed by the union of the splenic and superior mesenteric veins, but blood from the inferior mesenteric veins drains into the splenic vein before it merges with the superior mesenteric vein.

The reason for this detour of the blood through the liver before it returns to the heart will be further discussed in Chapter 6 (on the digestive system).

Table 4.1 (a) Arteries of the upper limbs

Artery	Origin	Branches
Brachiocephalic trunk (artery)	Arch of aorta	Right common carotid continuing as external and internal common carotid arteries (see Vol. 1, p. 46, Fig. 4.8 and Table 4.3 p. 47). Right subclavian
Subclavian	Brachiocephalic (right) Arch of aorta (left)	Two branches, i.e. vertebral artery supplying the brain and internal mammary artery supplying the breast. Enters the axillae and continues as axillary arteries
Axillary	Continuation of subclavian	Brachial artery running down medial aspect of upper arm and divides into radial and ulna arteries
Radial	Brachial	Palmar carpal, superficial palmar and dorsal carpal branches, deep palmar arch supplying lateral side of forearm, to the wrist and hand
Ulna	Brachial	Palmar carpal, dorsal carpal and deep palmar branches and superficial palmar arch supplying medial aspect of forearm to the wrist and hand

Table 4.1 (b) The aorta and its branches

Artery	Origin	Branches
Ascending aorta	Arising from left ventricle	Right and left coronary arteries, continuing as arch of aorta
Arch of aorta	Continuation of ascending aorta	Brachiocephalic trunk, left common carotid, left subclavian and continues as thoracic aorta
Descending thoracic aorta	Continuation of arch of aorta	Bronchial oesophageal, pericardiac and mediastinal branches, superior phrenic, posterior intercostal arteries (III–XI) and subcostal arteries, continues as abdominal aorta
Descending abdominal aorta	Left ventricle, lower portion of descending aorta	Inferior phrenic (diaphragm) coeliac which branches into gastric (stomach) splenic (pancreas and spleen) hepatic (liver, gall bladder, part of the stomach, duodenum and pancreas), right and left renal (kidneys) testicula (testes in the male), ovarian (ovaries in the female), superior mesenteric (small intestine), inferior mesenteric (large intestine); terminates in an inverted 'Y' formation to continue as right and left common iliac arteries

Table 4.1 (c) Arteries of the lower limbs

Artery	Origin	Branches
Right and left common iliac	Abdominal aorta	External and internal iliac arteries
External iliac	Common iliac	Inferior epigastric supplying the abdominal wall and external genitalia and runs obliquely downwards, behind the inguinal ligament, into the thigh to continue as the femoral artery
Internal iliac	Common iliac	Ilolumbar, obturator, superior gluteal, uterine, etc., to supply wall and viscera of pelvis, buttocks, reproductive organs and medial aspect of thigh
Femoral	Continuation of external iliac	From inguinal ligament extends downwards, anterior and medial surface of the thigh to enter popliteal space where it becomes the popliteal artery
Popliteal	Continuation of femoral	Lateral and medial genicular, anterior and posterior tibial, to supply knee and calf
Tibial anterior	Popliteal	Continues forward between tibia and fibula covering anterior aspect of ankle and foot to continue as dorsalis pedis
Tibial posterior	Popliteal	Continues downwards and medially and the branch near its origin, called the peroneal artery covers the lateral aspect of the leg. These arteries supply the leg and foot (including the heel) and continue as the plantar artery
Dorsalis pedis	Continuation of tibial anterior	Lateral and medial tarsal and arcuate arteries to supply foot including toes
Plantar	Tibial posterior	Deep and superficial branches supply muscles and joints of the foot, skin of the medial aspect of the sole and toes

N.B. For diagrams of the arteries of the lower leg, see Vol. 1, p. 229, Fig. 23.5.

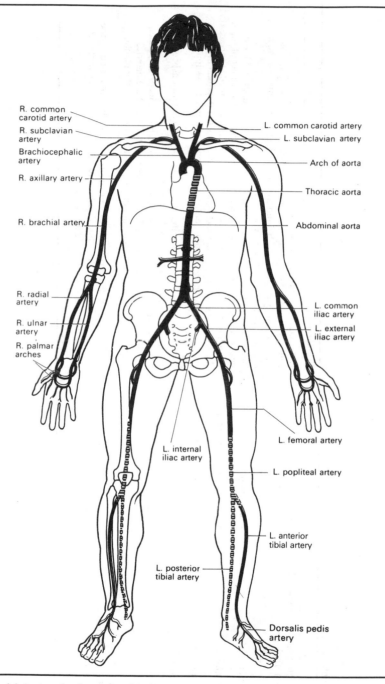

Fig. 4.6 Aorta and main arteries of the limbs

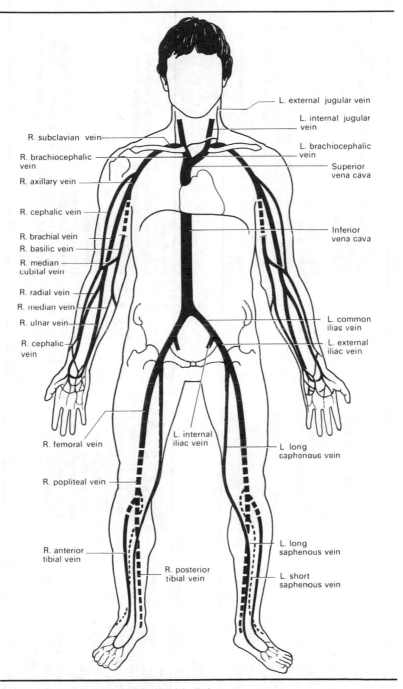

Fig. 4.7 Venae cavae and the main veins of the limbs

L. external jugular vein

L. internal jugular vein

R. subclavian vein

L. brachiocephalic vein

R. brachiocephalic vein

Superior vena cava

R. axillary vein

R. cephalic vein

Inferior vena cava

R. brachial vein

R. basilic vein

R. median cubital vein

R. radial vein

R. median vein

R. ulnar vein

L. common iliac vein

R. cephalic vein

L. external iliac vein

R. femoral vein

L. internal iliac vein

L. long saphenous vein

R. popliteal vein

R. anterior tibial vein

L. long saphenous vein

R. posterior tibial vein

L. short saphenous vein

Table 4.2 (a) Veins of the upper limbs

Vein	Region	Drains into
Ulna	Accompanies ulna artery	Joins radial veins at elbow to form brachial veins
Radial	Accompanies radial artery	Brachial veins
Cephalic	Anterior border of brachio-radial muscle and above elbow to lateral border of biceps muscle	Axillary vein
Median	Medial side of forearm	Basilic vein
Medial cubital	Connecting tributary from cephalic vein	Basilic vein
Basilic	Forearm	Joins brachial vein to form axillary vein
Brachial	Accompanies brachial artery	Joins basilic vein to form axillary vein
Axillary	Upper arm	At lateral border of first rib, becomes subclavian vein
Brachiocephalic	Thorax	Unite to form superior vena cava
Subclavian	Follows subclavian artery	Joins internal jugular vein for form brachiocephalic vein

Table 4.2 (b) Veins of the lower limbs

Vein	Region	Drains into
Tibial anterior	Follows tibial anterior artery	Joins tibial posterior vein to form popliteal vein
Tibial posterior	Follows tibial posterior artery	Joins tibial anterior vein to form popliteal vein
Long saphenous	Extends from dorsum of foot to just below inguinal ligament	Femoral vein
Short saphenous	Back of ankle and leg	Popliteal vein
Popliteal	Follows popliteal artery	Femoral vein
Femoral	Follows femoral artery covering two-thirds of thigh	External iliac vein
External iliac	Extends from the inguinal ligament to sacroiliac joint	Joins internal iliac vein to form common iliac vein
Internal iliac	Extends from sciatic notch to the brim of the pelvis	Joins external iliac vein to form common iliac vein
Common iliac	Ascends to right side of fifth lumbar vertebra	Unites with vein from other side to form inferior vena cava

NB For diagrams of the veins of the lower leg, see Vol. 1., p. 230 Fig. 23.7

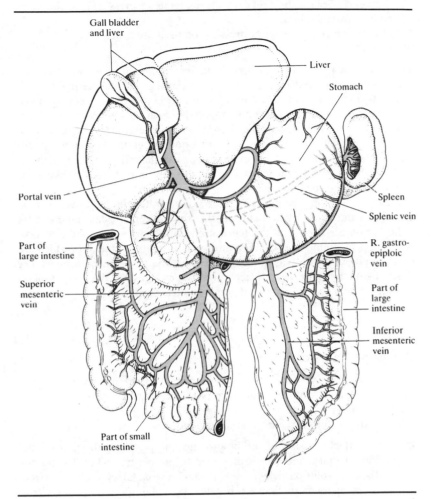

Fig. 4.8 Venous drainage from the abdominal organs and the formation of the portal vein

Varicose veins

Varicose veins are swollen, distended and knotted veins visible especially in the legs. The veins most commonly affected are the long and short saphenous veins and the tibial anterior vein and usually result from a stagnated or sluggish flow of the blood, probably in combination with defective valves and weakened walls of the veins. Varicose veins can occur due to:

● clients who must stand or sit motionless for long periods of time;

● age, whereby with increasing age, there is a progressive loss of elasticity in the vein walls;

● pregnancy, as more force is often necessary to push the blood through

the veins because the pregnant uterus tends to press against the veins coming from the legs;
● obesity, which puts a heavy pressure on the veins; and
● heredity.

The development of varicose veins is usually gradual; the client may have the feeling of heavy, tired legs and cramp in the legs during the night. As a beauty therapist you can offer advice in mild cases of varicose veins. Prevention is obviously better than treatment and those clients who have a predisposition to varicose veins should be advised to take regular leg exercises or long walks as these will stimulate the flow of blood through the legs; avoid standing or sitting for long periods of time; suggest that they make a point of walking about at frequent intervals and also advise that tight stockings or garters should not be worn.

Treatment can only be given by the medical profession but advice can be given to encourage the client to take rest periods during the day and use these to lie flat on the back with the feet raised slightly above the body; to take brief walks to stimulate circulation and suggest tights or stockings which are *lightly* reinforced with elastic to help support the veins in the legs. Heavy elastic tights/stockings, if not fitted correctly, may restrict the flow of blood and should only be recommended under medical supervision.

The lymphatic system

This system is actually a specialised component of the circulatory system, since it consists of a moving fluid (lymph) which is derived from the blood and tissue fluid.

The body contains three main kinds of fluid, i.e.

● blood, which consists of the blood cells and platelets, the plasma and various chemical substances dissolved in the plasma; when the plasma (without its solid particles) seeps through the capillary walls and circulates among the body tissues it is called tissue fluid;
● tissue fluid – when this fluid is drained from the tissues and collected by the lymphatic system, it is then called lymph;
● lymph, which is an odourless fluid, slightly alkaline, about 95 per cent water, containing a high concentration of lymphocytes.

A group of vessels, namely lymphatics, eventually return the lymph to the blood.

Lymphatic capillaries and vessels

Lying in the cellular spaces is the network of lymph vessels which begin as colourless blind-ended lymphatic capillaries which drain off excess tissue fluids and carry away waste material (see Fig. 4.9). These capillaries are composed of a very fine connective tissue and a single layer of endothelial

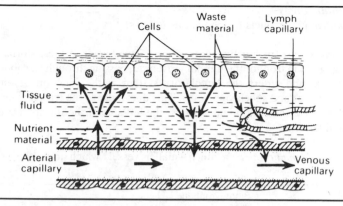

Fig. 4.9 Diagram of the beginning of a lymph capillary

cells and from these capillaries the lymph is carried into larger lymphatic vessels.

The structure of the lymphatic vessels consists of an outer coat of fibrous tissue, a middle coat of muscular and elastic tissue and an inner lining composed of a single layer of endothelial cells. The lymphatic vessels contain many semilunar valves which give them a knotted appearance and these prevent the backward flow of lymph (see Fig. 4.10). The lymph in the vessels is moved onwards by the contraction of the surrounding muscles and aided by the presence of valves in some of the larger lymphatic channels. As lymph vessels become larger they join together, eventually forming two ducts.

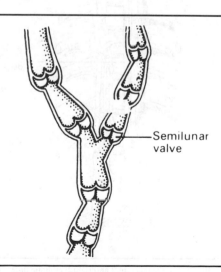

Fig. 4.10 A lymph vessel cut open to show semilunar valves

Lymphatic ducts
The two lymphatic ducts formed are as follows.

The thoracic duct (or left lymphatic duct)   This begins in the cisterna chyli (see Fig. 4.11) in front of the lumbar vertebrae, passing through the abdomen and thorax, and enters the circulatory system at the junction of the left internal jugular and subclavian veins. This duct collects the lymph from both legs, the pelvic and abdominal cavities, the left side of the thorax, head and neck and left arm.

The right lymphatic duct   a much smaller vessel, which joins the venous

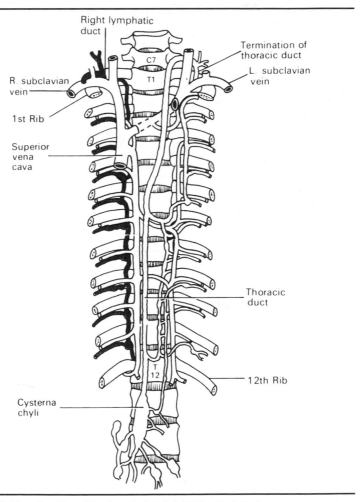

Fig. 4.11 Origin and position of the thoracic duct and right lymphatic duct

system at the junction of the right internal jugular and subclavian veins and collects lymph from the right side of the head and neck, the right side of the thorax and right arm (see Fig. 4.11 and Fig. 4.12).

Lymphatic nodes

Lymphatic nodes (or glands) have been described in detail in Vol. 1, Chap. 17, p. 165; Figure 17.1 (Vol. 1) shows a section through a lymph node, and Fig. 17.2 (Vol. 1) show some of the lymph nodes of the face and neck. The main groups of nodes lie in the neck, axilla, thorax, abdomen and groin and Table 4.3 details the areas where the lymph is drained through the relevant nodes.

For the positions of these nodes see Fig. 4.13 showing some of the lymph nodes of the upper limb and Fig. 4.14, the lymph nodes of the lower limb.

In beauty therapy the importance of learning these nodes is paramount when effecting lymphatic drainage massage or vacuum massage where the objective is to assist the removal of waste products through the lymphatic system.

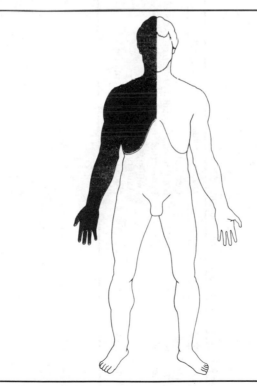

Fig. 4.12 Diagram of lymph drainage. Dark area drained by the thoracic duct. Light area drained by the right lymphatic duct

Table 4.3 Lymph drainage through relevant nodes

Lymph from:	Drains through the following nodes:
Head and neck	Cervical
Upper limbs	Supratrochlear, axillary (deep and superficial)
Thoracic cavity	Parasternal, intercostal, brachiocephalic, mediastinal, tracheobronchial, bronchopulmonary, oesphageal
Breast	Axillary
Abdominal and pelvis	Numerous nodes to cisterna chyli
Lower limbs	Popliteal, inguinal

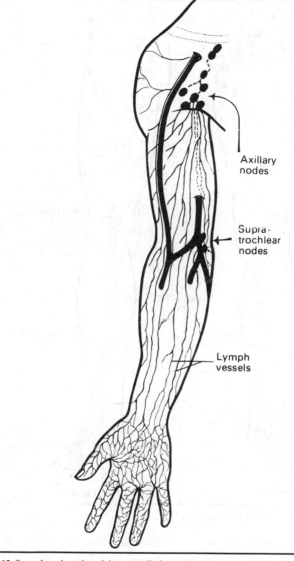

Fig. 4.13 Some lymph nodes of the upper limb

Lymphatic organs
There are larger masses of lymphatic tissue called lymphatic organs and these include the spleen, tonsils and thymus.

The spleen   is a large purplish gland lying on the left side of the abdomen beneath the 9th, 10th and 11th ribs. It touches the left kidney, the splenic

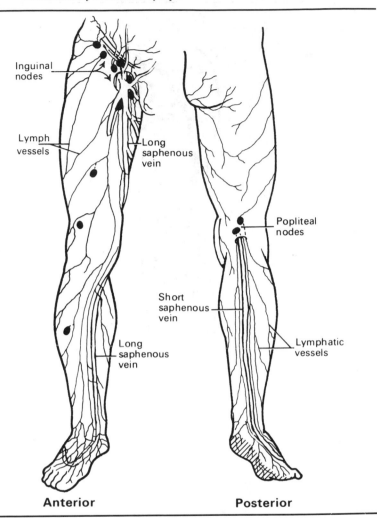

Fig. 4.14 Some lymph nodes of the lower limb

flexure of the colon and the tail of the pancreas. The spleen contains lymphoid tissue, manufactures lymphocytes and also has phagocytes which remove worn-out red cells and other foreign bodies in the bloodstream. It also converts haemoglobin to bilirubin and releases iron into the blood for further use.

The tonsils   are also composed of lymph tissue and there are three different kinds, i.e.

● palatine tonsils, a pair of oval-shaped structures, partially embedded in the mucous membrane, one on each side of the back of the throat;

● lingual tonsils, which lie at the base of the tongue, and
● pharyngeal tonsils (or adenoids) which lie on the wall of the nasal part of the pharynx.

These help to filter the circulating lymph of bacteria and any other foreign material that may enter the body, especially through the nose and the mouth.

The thymus   is a two-lobed ductless gland situated behind the thorax and extending to the neck. Its exact functions are unknown but it is believed to be concerned with the production of antibodies.

Disorders of the lymphatic system

Lymphadenitis is an inflammation of the lymph nodes, particularly in the neck, e.g. swollen tonsils. Lymphangitis is the inflammation of a lymphatic vessel. However, it is unlikely that the beauty therapist will come into contact with disorders of the lymphatic system.

Chapter 5

Respiratory system

Respiration is the exchange of oxygen and carbon dioxide in the body, i.e. in the lungs, between the cell and its environment, and in the metabolism of the cell.

The respiratory system is the group of organs whose function it is to provide for the transfer of oxygen from the air to the blood and of waste carbon dioxide from the blood to the air. The sequence of the respiration process begins as air enters the nose or mouth passing through the pharynx, the larynx (known as the upper respiratory tract) and the trachea and into the bronchi and the lungs (known as the lower respiratory tract) (see Fig. 5.1).

Upper respiratory tract

The nose

The nose has three main functions:

- provides a natural pathway by which air enters the body by breathing;
- acts as a protective device; and
- is the organ of smell.

The external part of the nose consists of bone and cartilage. The two nasal bones project downwards and also form the bridge between the eyes. The nasal cartilages and the cartilages of the nostrils give the shape and firmness of the nose. The nostrils lead into two nasal cavities which are separated from each other by the nasal septum. The interior of the nose is lined with very vascular *ciliated columnar epithelium* (ciliated mucous membrane) and it is this which moistens and warms the air as it is inhaled and filters dust particles and other impurities.

Three ridges of bone (the turbinate bones) project from the outer wall of each nasal cavity and partially divide the cavity into three air passages and at the back of the nose these passages lead to the pharynx.

The pharynx

The pharynx is a tube about 5 in (12–13 cm) long lying behind the nasal

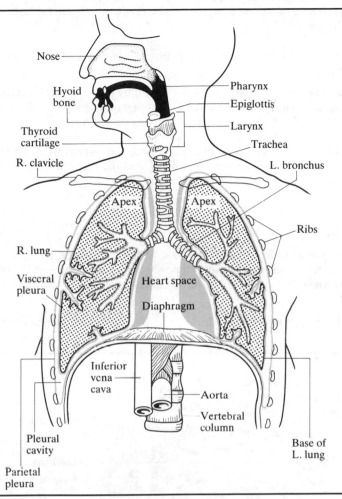

Fig. 5.1 The organs of respiration

cavities, mouth and larynx and communicating with them and with the oesophagus. It is divided into three parts:

The nasopharynx   lies behind the nose above the level of the soft palate. It provides a passage for air during breathing and it also contains the openings of the Eustachian tubes through which air enters the middle ear.

   At the back of the nasal cavity and above the mouth lie two bodies of lymph tissue called the pharyngeal tonsils. Infection and enlargement of this tissue may cause adenoids and prevent nasal breathing.

The oropharynx   lies behind the mouth but below the level of the soft palate. The palatine and lingual tonsils occur on the lateral walls of the oropharynx.

The laryngopharynx   extends from the oropharynx and continues as the oesophagus.

The pharynx is separated from the mouth by the soft palate and its fleshy V-shaped extension called the *uvula*. During swallowing, the soft palate is raised, closing off the nasopharynx as food passes from the mouth to the oesophagus (see Fig. 5.2).

Therefore the pharynx is involved in both the respiratory system, by air passing through the nasal and oral parts, and the digestive system by food passing through the oral and laryngeal parts.

The larynx

The larynx is situated below the root of the tongue and hyoid bone and extends to the trachea, providing a passageway for air between the pharynx and trachea. It is composed of cartilages held together by muscles and ligaments, i.e.

● the *epiglottis* cartilage, which lies at the base of the tongue, closes the

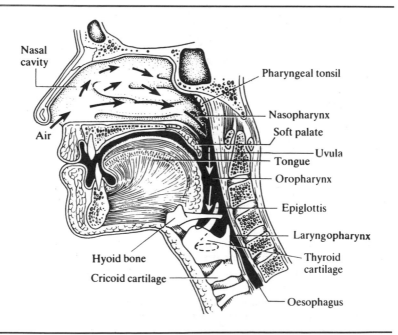

Fig. 5.2 Arrows showing the pathways of air from the nose to the larynx

larynx as it is lifted up during swallowing, so preventing the passage of food or drink into the larynx and trachea;

- the *thyroid* cartilage which forms a laryngeal prominence, i.e. the Adam's apple;
- the *cricoid* cartilage, which lies below the thyroid cartilage (shaped like a signet ring), surrounds the larynx and articulates posteriorly with
- the *arytenoid* cartilages; these give attachment to two flexible vocal cords which are manipulated by small muscles to produce sound as heard in speech and therefore the larynx is also called the *voice box* (see Fig. 5.3).

Infections of the upper respiratory tract include the common cold, influenza, pharyngitis, laryngitis and tonsilitis.

Lower respiratory tract

The trachea

The trachea (or windpipe) is the air passage extending from the throat and larynx to the main bronchi. This tube is about 4 in (10 cm) long and to keep the passage uniformly open, it is reinforced at the front and at the sides by a series of C-shaped rings of hyaline cartilage. Connective tissue and involuntary muscle join the cartilages and form the posterior wall where the rings are incomplete and this arrangement prevents any obstruction of the air passage when the head or neck move (see Fig. 5.4). The trachea is also lined with

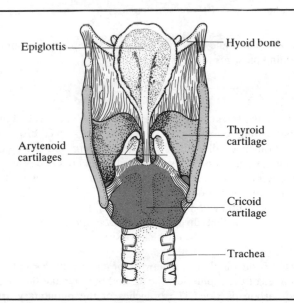

Epiglottis

Hyoid bone

Arytenoid
cartilages

Thyroid
cartilage

Cricoid
cartilage

Trachea

Fig. 5.3 Larynx – viewed from behind

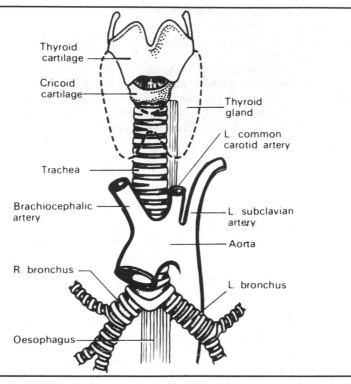

Thyroid cartilage

Cricoid cartilage

Thyroid gland

L. common carotid artery

Trachea

Brachiocephalic artery

L. subclavian artery

Aorta

R. bronchus

L. bronchus

Oesophagus

Fig. 5.4 The trachea and some of its associated structures

cilated mucous membrane which continuously sweep any foreign matter out of the breathing passages towards the mouth.

The bronchi

At its lower end the trachea divides into two smaller tubes called the *primary bronchi*, one leading to each lung. Within the lungs, each bronchus divides into smaller branches called the *secondary bronchi* and these continue to branch, forming small *bronchioles*. The trachea and the two primary bronchi and their many branches resemble an inverted tree trunk with its branches and are, therefore, spoken of as the bronchial tree (see Fig. 5.5).

The bronchioles subdivide into smaller tubes, terminating eventually into microscopic branches that divide into *alveolar ducts*, which terminate in several alveolar sacs, the walls of which consist of numerous *alveoli* (see Fig. 5.6).

Each alveoli is surrounded by a network of fine capillaries and through the thin membranes of the capillaries, the air and blood make their exchange of oxygen and carbon dioxide. The branches of the pulmonary artery carry carbon dioxide rich blood, and this gas is given up in return for the oxygen in the new air which has entered the alveolar sacs. The lungs then exhale the

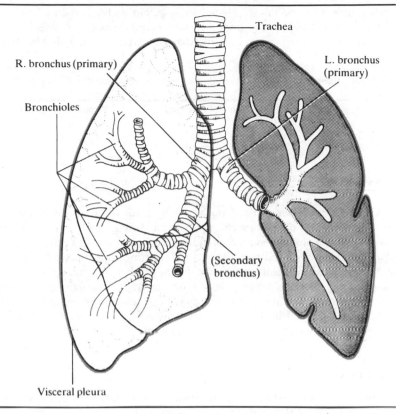

Fig. 5.5 The bronchial tree and the lungs. Anterior part of the left lung removed

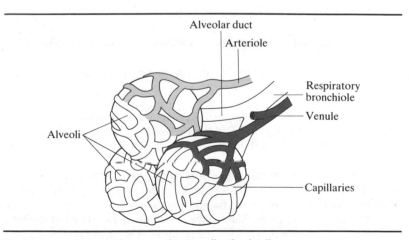

Fig. 5.6 Diagram of the capillary network surrounding the alveoli

carbon dioxide in the de-oxygenated air, together with a certain amount of water vapour, which comes from the moist membranes of the alveoli. The percentages of various gases in inspired and expired air is detailed in Table 5.1.

Table 5.1   *Composition of air (percentages of various gases in inspired and expired air)*

	% by volume of gases in air breathed in:	% by volume of gases in air breathed out:
Oxygen	21	17
Carbon dioxide	0.03	4
Water vapour	variable	increased
Nitrogen	78	78
Other gases	traces	traces

A bacterial infection of the bronchi usually leads to bronchitis and there are other diseases of the bronchi, i.e. asthma. Briefly, asthma is cramp or spasm of the involuntary muscles of the bronchi, obstructing the free passage of air. As these fibres contract they squeeze the tubes and impede the flow of air. There is extrinsic asthma which is due to an allergy to antigens; usually the offending allergens are suspended in the air but occasionally it is related to food or drugs. Intrinsic asthma is usually associated with recurrent infections of the bronchi, sinuses or tonsils and adenoids. This is mentioned here as it will obviously affect any exercise programme planned for the client.

The lungs

There are two lungs which are cone-shaped organs, large enough to fill the pleural portion of the thoracic cavity completely. They extend from the diaphragm to a point slightly above the clavicles and each lung is described as having an apex, a base, a costal surface and a medial surface.

The apex   is rounded and projects above the clavicle.

The base   is concave and semilunar in shape and rests on the diaphragm.

The costal surface   of each lung lies against the ribs and is rounded to match the contours of the thoracic cavity.

The medial surface   of each lung is roughly concave to allow room for the *mediastinum*, i.e. the area occupied by the heart, the great vessels, trachea, right and left bronchus, oesophagus, lymph nodes and vessels and nerves. (Some of the organs associated with the lungs are shown in Fig. 5.7.) The concavity is greater on the left than on the right because of the position of the heart. The primary bronchi and the pulmonary blood vessels (bound together by connective tissue to form what is known as the *root* of the lung) enter each lung through a slit on its medial surface called the *hilum*. Parts of the lung and some of the structures entering the hilum are shown in Fig. 5.8.

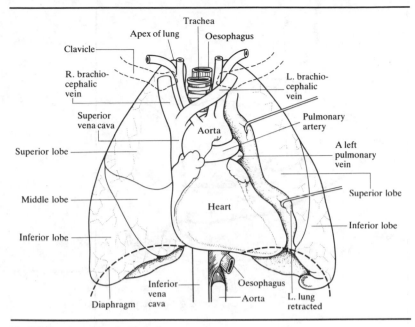

Fig. 5.7 Organs associated with the lungs

Each lung is divided into lobes by fissures. The left lung is divided into two lobes (superior and inferior) and the right lung into three lobes (superior, middle and inferior). Each secondary bronchus is named for the lung lobe it enters, i.e. the superior secondary bronchus enters the superior lobe etc.

Both lungs are enveloped by a double membranous bag or sac known as the *pleura*, i.e.

- the parietal pleura lines the thoracic cavity; and
- the visceral pleura adheres to the lung.

The pleural cavity is the very small space between the two membranes of the pleura which is filled with a very thin film of serous fluid to prevent friction between them during breathing (see Fig. 5.1).

Inspiration and expiration

Contraction of the diaphragm alone, or of the diaphragm and the external intercostal muscles, produces quiet inspiration. As the diaphragm contracts, it descends, making the thoracic cavity longer; also contraction of the external intercostal muscles pulls the anterior end of each rib up and outwards. In this way the thoracic cavity is enlarged from front to back and side to side letting air rush in (see Fig. 5.9).

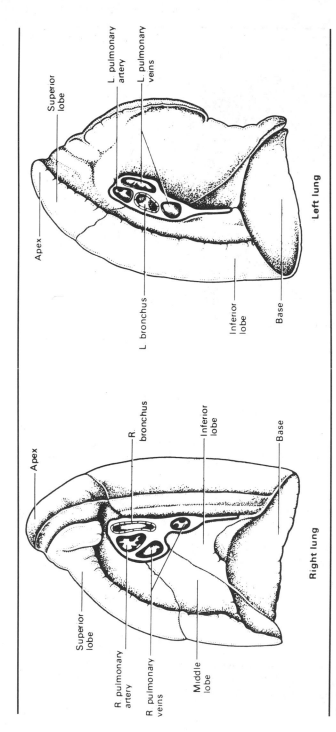

Fig. 5.8 The parts of the lungs and some structures entering at the hilum

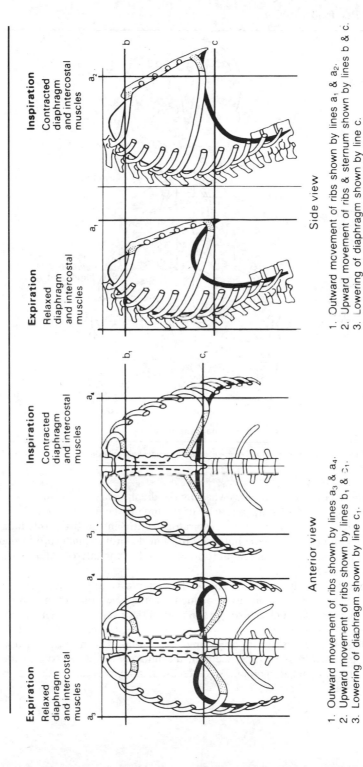

Expiration
Relaxed diaphragm and intercostal muscles

Inspiration
Contracted diaphragm and intercostal muscles

Anterior view

1. Outward movement of ribs shown by lines a_3 & a_4.
2. Upward movement of ribs shown by lines b_1 & c_1.
3. Lowering of diaphragm shown by line c_1.

Expiration
Relaxed diaphragm and intercostal muscles

Inspiration
Contracted diaphragm and intercostal muscles

Side view

1. Outward movement of ribs shown by lines a_1 & a_2.
2. Upward movement of ribs & sternum shown by lines b & c.
3. Lowering of diaphragm shown by line c.

Fig. 5.9 Diagram of the changes in capacity of the thoracic cavity (and the lungs) during breathing

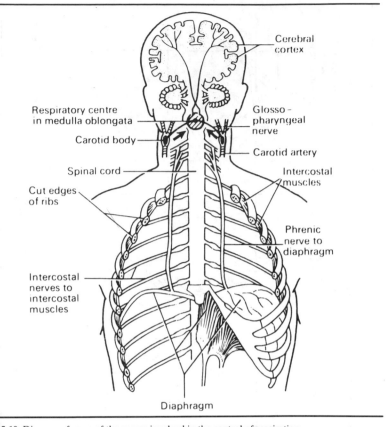

Fig. 5.10 Diagram of some of the nerves involved in the control of respiration

Expiration is a passive process whereby the diaphragm and the intercostal muscles relax and the natural elasticity of the lung tissue forces air out.

Breathing is controlled by the respiratory centre in the brain (medulla oblongata and pons) whereby impulses are sent down the spinal cord to the nerves that control the diaphragm (phrenic), and to the intercostal muscles (intercostal) (see Fig. 5.10).

Chemical and reflex signals control these nerve centres. The chemical controls of breathing are mainly dependent on the levels of carbon dioxide rather than the amount of oxygen present. For instance, if there is an increase in carbon dioxide due to physical exercise, the brain will respond and adjust the breathing rate accordingly. Breathing becomes deeper and more rapid in response to the needs of the muscles for more oxygen; the heartbeat is stimulated, blood flow is increased and excess carbon dioxide is breathed out.

Chapter 6

Nutrition and the digestive system

Nutrition

Nutrition is particularly concerned with those properties of food that build sound bodies and promote health. A basic knowledge of this subject will assist the beauty therapist to advise clients of a balanced diet, which contains adequate amounts of the essential nutritional elements that the body must have to function normally.

The essential ingredients of a balanced diet are:

carbohydrates
● proteins
● fats
● vitamins
mineral elements
● water.

Carbohydrates

They are present, at least in small quantities, in most foods, but the chief sources are the sugars and starches found in foods such as sugar, jam, fruit, vegetables, including potatoes, cereals, bread, biscuits, rice and wheat. A carbohydrate is a compound of carbon, hydrogen and oxygen and is classified, according to its chemical composition, as either a monosaccharide, disaccharide or polysaccharide.

A monosaccharide is a simple sugar; examples include glucose, fructose and galactose:

glucose is found naturally in ripe fruits, honey and in some vegetables e.g. onions; during digestion and metabolism carbohydrates are converted to glucose which is then used as a main energy source in the body;
● *fructose* is sweeter than glucose and is also found in fruits and honey;
galactose is formed during digestion of lactose or milk sugar.

Disaccharides consist of two monosaccharide molecules chemically combined to form sugars. For example:

● *sucrose*, found in cane and beet sugar, yields glucose and fructose;
maltose, or malt sugar, is produced during digestion of cooked starch, each molecule yields two glucose molecules;
lactose, or milk sugar, is found in all types of milk, yielding glucose and galactose.

A polysaccharide   yields ten or more monosaccharides. The most important examples are starch and cellulose:

Starch is present in the form of granules in the cells of plants, such as cereals, potatoes and root vegetables and acts as a reserve store of food for the plant itself. Starch is released from the granules during cooking.
Glycogen is a type of starch (animal) formed in the body from glucose and stored in the liver and muscles as a future energy source.
Cellulose (roughage) is a fibrous polysaccharide forming cell walls of plants, e.g. fruit and vegetable fibres, bran from cereal grains. The human body cannot digest this type of polysaccharide but it forms roughage or dietary fibre, adding bulk to the diet and stimulating intestinal evacuation. An inadequate supply of roughage may lead to gastrointestinal disorders.

If carbohydrates are eaten in excessive amounts, the body changes them into fat and stores them in that way.

To summarise, the functions of carbohydrates are:

to provide energy for physical and mental exertion;
to supply immediate calories and so save on protein;
to assist in the assimilation and digestion of other foods.

Proteins

A protein is a compound containing carbon, hydrogen, oxygen, nitrogen and may contain sulphur and/or phosphorus, the characteristic element being nitrogen. Protein compounds are built up of smaller molecules called *amino acids* and these are divided into two categories, i.e.

essential amino acids which cannot be synthesised in the body and therefore must be included in a diet.
non-essential amino acids which can be synthesised in the body.

Protein foods that provide large amounts of essential amino acids are known as *complete* proteins and these include proteins found in meat, fish, eggs, milk and soya beans. Proteins that cannot supply the body with all the essential amino acids are known as *incomplete* proteins and these can be found in peas, beans, lentils, (pulses) other vegetables, nuts and certain forms of wheat.

Proteins are essential to life, they:

● build and repair body tissue;
● satisfy hunger;
● have the ability to build hormones and enzymes which aid in energy production;
● aid digestion of food and excretion;
● make haemoglobin within the red corpuscles;
● assist in the clotting of the blood;
● form antibodies to fight infection and disease.

When excess protein is consumed, over and above the body's needs, the nitrogenous part is separated and excreted by the kidneys and the rest is usually stored as fat in the cells of adipose tissue.

Fats

Fats consist of carbon, hydrogen and oxygen in various chemical combinations. Fats are divided into two groups *animal* and *vegetable*.

Animal fat is found in milk, butter, eggs, cheese, meat and oily fish, such as herring, cod and halibut, all of which contain *saturated* fatty acids and glycerol (glycerin) and are solid at room temperature.

Vegetable fat is found in soft margarine and in vegetable oils, i.e. olive oil, containing *unsaturated* (also called *polyunsaturated*) fatty acids and glycerol and are liquid at room temperature.

The functions of fats are to:

● provide a delayed source of energy;
● act as carriers for fat-soluble vitamins (A, D, E and K);
● prevent the skin from becoming dry (i.e. secretions of the sebaceous glands);
● protect vital organs of the body, i.e. kidneys and eyes;
● form a fatty layer under the skin to preserve heat and protect the body against cold.

Cholesterol is a fatty or oily substance which normally forms part of the wall around each cell in the body. However, when it becomes lodged in the walls of arteries, it contributes to atherosclerosis which in turn causes heart attacks or strokes. This is mentioned here as it is thought that the saturated fats found in animal fat seem to increase cholesterol levels whereas unsaturated fats from vegetable sources do not. For interest, Table 6.1 gives a diet plan for the lowering of cholesterol levels.

Vitamins

Vitamins are organic substances found in *foods* and are essential in small quantities for growth and good health. They are divided into two main groups: those soluble in fat (A, D, E and K) which enable them to be stored

Table 6.1 Diet plan for the lowering of cholesterol levels

This diet plan is moderate in fat and cholesterol content with minimal amounts of those saturated fats which may elevate blood cholesterol level. It has a high fibre content and carbohydrate foods should preferably be eaten in their unrefined state (e.g. fresh fruit rather than fruit juice)

Serving size depends on activity level and body weight. If overweight, limit serving size, also limit all types of fat and oil and increase physical activity.

Sodium intake should be restricted to less than 2000 mg sodium per day. This is equivalent to 1 tsp or 5 gm of salt, *including* the natural sodium in foods. Remember that sodium is widely distributed in foods and frequently added in processing and packaging. Check food labels for salt or sodium compounds.

Breakfast:	Select from the following:	
	Fruit,	fresh, whole in preference to juice
	Cereal,	muesli – puffed wheat – rice – wheatgerm – bran – Weetabix – porridge, plus skimmed milk or yoghurt (low fat) or diluted apple juice
	Egg,	2 to 3 eggs allowed weekly, boiled or poached
	Cottage cheese, with bread, crackers, fruit, salad, etc.	
	Nuts, seeds, peanut paste, (limit if overweight) tomatoes, mushrooms, onions, salads etc.	
	Bread,	wholegrain, toast, crispbreads, crackers, with polyunsaturated margarine
	Drinks,	water, fruit juice, tea, coffee, skim milk
Lunch:	Choose from the following:	
	Soup,	fresh vegetable soup which may contain rice, barley, lentils, or other grains or pulses
	Salad,	a variety of any salad vegetables, including bean or seed sprouts use avocado, dried and fresh fruits, nuts, seeds, grains, pulses, etc. to add variety to salads. Also use fresh herbs, especially parsley.
		dressing, use lemon juice or polyunsaturated oil with lemon juice or cider vinegar
	Cottage cheese, fish, pulses (not canned)	
	Nuts, seeds, peanut paste,	
	Jacket potato, wholemeal bread or crispbread, dark rye bread, cooked wholegrains	
	Fruit,	fresh, dried or stewed
	Drinks,	water, diluted fruit juice, mineral water, herb teas

Dinner: Choose from the
             following
             Soup,   fat free; vegetables, beans
             Meat,   small to moderate serving of lean meat (3–4 oz or 100 gm)
                             cut away all visible fat. Avoid offal meats
             or
             Chicken   quarter of chicken, remove all skin, white meat has less fat
             or
             Fish   average serving of fish (use polyunsaturated oil if frying)
             or
             Vegetarian dish, using dry beans, peas, nuts, seeds, wholegrains, vegetables
             Potatoes, brown rice, wholemeal pasta,
             Vegetables and or salad
             Fruit,   fresh
             Drinks,   water, mineral water, tea, coffee, wine or alcohol in moderation (1–2 glasses)

Note: Meat and chicken should not be taken more than three times weekly.

Between meals: Fresh fruit, raw vegetables,
                Nuts, seeds, dried fruit,
                Yoghurt (low fat)
                Bread (wholemeal) or crispbreads (with polyunsaturated margarine)
                Drinks, water, tea, coffee, coffee substitute, herb teas, diluted fruit juices, mineral water etc.

Note: If overweight, avoid eating between meals.

Table 6.2 Fat-soluble vitamins – A, D, E, and K

Vitamins	Food source	Function	Deficiency results in:	Destroyed by:	Max. daily dose
A (Retinol)	Apricots Asparagus Avocado pears Bananas Beans, (French, runner, broad) Broccoli Brussel sprouts Butter Cabbage Carrots Cheese Cherries Cod liver oil Cream Eggs Green peppers Kidneys Liver Margarine Milk Parsley Peaches Peas Prunes Spinach Spring greens Sweet potatoes Tomatoes Turnip tops Watercress	Healthy complexion Good eyesight Regeneration of the visual purple in the retina of the eye Protects surface tissues of the respiratory tract Helps repair body tissues and skeletal growth	Dryness and premature ageing of the skin Night blindness Inflammation of the eyes Aggravation of the respiratory tract	Exposure to sunlight. Air pollution i.e. smoke and smog	5000 i.u.

Vitamin	Sources	Function	Deficiency symptoms	Enemies	Amount
D (Calciferol)	Butter Cheese Cod liver oil Eggs Herrings Mackerel Milk Sardines Tinned salmon	Encourages the transport of calcium and phosphorous to tissues which build bones and teeth	Softening of the bones Curvature of the spine Muscle cramp Pain in the joints Tooth decay Arteriosclerosis Rickets in children but very rare	Air pollution i.e. smoke and smog	400 i.u.
E (Tocopherol)	Apples Asparagus Blackberries Cabbage Carrots Celery Cod liver oil Cod's roe Eggs Leeks Muesli Olive oil Parsley Rolled oats Sunflower seeds/oil Tomatoes Tuna fish Wheatgerm Wholemeal bread	Unites with oxygen to protect red blood cells. Counteracts the process of ageing. Externally used for burns, bruises and wounds to accelerate healing. Maintains healthy muscular system	Early onset of old age. Sluggish circulation. Varicose veins. Abnormal fat deposits in muscles	Cooking and storage	20 i.u.
K	Broccoli Brussel sprouts Cabbage Cauliflower Eggs Oats Potatoes Strawberries Wheat germ Yoghurt	Helps liver to produce substances important in blood clotting. Prevents haemorrhaging	Slows blood clotting Haemorrhaging	Alcohol Light Sulphur Antibodies	Negligible

Table 6.3. Water-soluble vitamins – B Complex and C

Vitamins	Food source dose	Function	Deficiency results	Destroyed	Max. daily dose
B1 (Thiamine)	Alfafa sprouts Asparagus Bacon Beef Brazil nuts Brewer's yeast Brown rice Eggs Haricot beans Lamb Liver Milk Peanuts Peas Pork Potatoes Wheatgerm Wholemeal bread	Necessary for the conversion of carbohydrates into glucose for energy. Helps to regulate smooth function of nervous system, heart and liver. Associated with the control of water balance in the body.	Loss of appetite and stamina. Fatigue Forgetfulness Certain types of neuritis. (Beriberi – very rare)	Cooking, Soaking Alcohol Tobacco	1.5 mg
B2 (Riboflavin)	Almonds Avocado pears Beans Beef Brewer's yeast Cottage cheese Kidney Lamb Milk Mushrooms Peas Pork Rabbit	Promotes growth and general health. Required for cell respiration and tissue repair. Concerned with the oxidation of all foods. Necessary for good vision and clear eyes. Associated with the physiology of the skin.	Broken blood vessels. Bloodshot and itching eyes. Sensitivity to bright light. Seborrhoeic dermatitis Dandruff. Open sores at the corners of the mouth and on the lips. Split finger nails.	Light Alkalis	2 mg

Vitamin	Sources	Function	Deficiency symptoms	Destroyed by	Amount
B 2 (contd)	Spinach Wheatgerm Wholemeal bread Yoghurt				
B3 (Niacin or Nicotinic acid)	Beef Chicken Dried peas Halibut Kidneys Lamb Liver Mackerel Peanuts Pork Salmon Sardines Tuna fish Turkey Wheatgerm Wholemeal bread	Acts to utilise carbohydrates, fats and amino acids Important to mental health. Maintains health of skin, tongue, gums and digestive system	Pellagra (i.e. various skin, digestive and mental disturbances). Halitosis. Dental decay, Lethargy		15 mg
B5 (Pantothenic acid)	Bran Brewer's yeast Kidneys Liver Mushrooms Peanuts Wholegrains	Associated in the metabolism of fats and carbohydrates. Important for nerves, stress and digestion	Fatigue. Headaches. Disturbance of sleep. Irritability. Nausea. Premature grey hair. Early onset of arthritis	Acid (i.e. vinegar) Heat. Freezing	5.10 mg
B6 (Pyridoxine)	Bananas Bran Brazil nuts Chicken Eggs Liver Mackerel Walnuts Wheatgerm Wholemeal bread	Essential for metabolism of certain amino acids and for cellular function. Regulation of the nervous system. Helps to form collagen and elastin to keep skin firm and smooth	These are rare:– Inflammation of the nerves Irritability Anaemia Muscle weakness Seborrhoeic or inflammation of the skin	Oral contraceptives Some amount by soaking or cooking of food.	2 mg

contd

Vitamins	Food source dose	Function	Deficiency results	Destroyed	Max. daily dose
B12 (Cyano-cobalamin)	Beef Cheese Cod Egg yolks Haddock Herrings Kidneys Liver Milk Oysters Rabbit Sardines Soya beans Tuna fish	Needed for efficient production of blood cells and for the health of the nervous system	Pernicious anaemia Disturbance of the central nervous system. Unpleasant body odour	Heat Foods in conjunction with raw egg white	0.005 mg
Biotin (vit. B Complex)	Blackcurrants Cauliflower Dried milk Egg Yolks Kidneys Leeks Liver Rolled oats Tomatoes	Helps to form fatty acids and assimulates these with carbohydrates for energy. Growth of bacteria	Possible fatigue and depression. Loss of good colour of the skin. Dermatitis Conjunctivitis	Exposure to air. Baking soda Raw egg whites	0.003 mg
Choline (vit. B Complex)	Beans Fish Heart Lecithin granules Lentils Wheatgerm Wholegrains	Desaturates fats from the liver	In rare cases: Cirrhosis of the liver Arteriosclerosis High blood pressure	Strong alkali	Negligible

Vitamin	Food sources	Function	Deficiency symptoms	Destroyed by	Recommended daily amount
Folic acid (vit. B Complex)	Almonds, Advocado pears, Beetroot, Bran, Brewer's yeast, Cauliflower, Chicory, Cod, Cucumber, Hazelnuts, Lemon juice, Lettuce, Liver, Cranges, Cysters, Peanuts, Peas, Potatoes, Spinach, Sweetcorn, Walnuts, Wheat	Essential for maturation of erythrocytes in the red bone marrow. Significant in age retardation	Anaemia, Depression, Ageing	Heat, Moisture	0.002 mg
Inositol (vit. B Complex)	Bran, Lecithin granules, Nuts, Oats, Sesame seeds, Wheatgerm	Together with choline, necessary for the formation of lecithin to desaturate fats from the liver	Poor appetite, Cirrhosis of the liver, Arteriosclerosis	*	Negligible
Paba (Para-aminobenzoic acid) (vit. B Complex)	Broccoli, Brown rice, Cabbage, Kale, Kidneys, Liver	Together with other 'B' vitamins, helps to form red blood cells	Fatigue, Depression, Digestive disorders	*	Negligible

contd

Vitamins	Food source	Function	Deficiency results	Destroyed	Max. daily dose
	dose				
C (Ascorbic acid)	Asparagus Avocado pears Bananas Blackcurrants Broad beans Broccoli Brussel sprouts Cabbage Cauliflower Grapefruit Leeks Lemon juice Lettuce Liver Melon Onions Oranges Parsley Parsnips Plantain Peppers Pineapple Potatoes Radishes Raspberries Spinach Spring greens Strawberries Tangerines Tomatoes Turnips Watercress	Essential to bone tissue, collagen formation, vascular function, tissue respiration and wound healing. Produces antibodies Counteracts stress	Haemorrhaging Tendency to bruise or bleed and slow to heal. Gingivitis Tooth decay Poor vision In rare cases – scurvy	Light Heat Excess cooking Storage Acids Alkalis	50 mg

in the body for future use, and those soluble in water (C and B complex) which must be replaced every day, as any excess is excreted through the urine. These are detailed in Tables 6.2 and 6.3. It is important to remember that the body requires vitamins just as it requires other food constituents, i.e. carbohydrates, proteins, fats, mineral elements and water.

Mineral elements

These are inorganic substances required for all body processes. Listed in Table 6.4 are the major mineral elements and Table 6.5 are the minor mineral elements or trace elements. These mineral elements occur in the body in very small quantities but are essential to many metabolic processes. Many act like catalysts and when their work is done they are excreted in the urine and sweat, which means that they have to be replaced regularly from natural sources. Normally, mineral requirements are satisfied by a varied or mixed diet of animal and vegetable products which meet the energy and protein needs.

Water

Water is a colourless liquid compound of two parts hydrogen and one part oxygen. Our bodies are about two-thirds water and normally the level remains fairly constant.

Water enters the body from the digestive tract, in the liquids drunk and the foods eaten. It is also produced by each body cell during catabolism of foods and this water enters the bloodstream. Therefore, water is needed for the functioning of every organ in the body; it aids circulation, digestion, absorption, excretion and regulation of body temperature. Normally, the total volume of water entering the body equals the total volume leaving the body via the kidneys (urine), lungs (water in expired air), skin (by diffusion and sweat) and the intestines (faeces).

Diet

The principle of all diets should be based on the balance of food intake and energy output. Nutritional food values must be taken into consideration for any type of diet and advice can be given to avoid foods that have a low nutrient value, i.e.

- refined sugar, sweets, confectionary;
- refined breads and biscuits, refined cereals, pasta, white rice, cakes, pastries and puddings;
- cordials and soft drinks; and
- a high intake of fried foods or processed foods should also be avoided.

Table 6.4 Major mineral elements

Mineral	Food source	Function	Deficiency results in:	Daily need
Calcium	Almonds Black treacle Bran Brazil nuts Broccoli Clams Dried figs Hard cheese Haricot beans Milk Mussels Parsley Pilchards Sardines Sesame seeds Shrimps Spinach Sprats Watercress Yoghurt	Together with vitamin D and phosphorous it is needed for the hardening of the teeth and formation of bone. It is also needed for the maintenance of the heart beat, clotting of blood and normal functioning of muscles and nerves	Bones and teeth softening. Impaired blood clotting. Muscular disturbances i.e. cramp. Nervous disturbances i.e. numbness and tingling in arms and legs	600–1000 mg
Chlorine	Carrots Celery Fish Lettuce Meat Milk Salt Spinach Tomatoes Watercress	Usually related to sodium levels in the tissues and is concerned with cell metabolism	(Deficiency unlikely to occur)	Trace

| Iron | 18 mg | Essential for the formation of haemoglobin in the red corpuscles. Also necessary for tissue oxidation | Black treacle
Bran
Brazil nuts
Cocoa
Curry powder
Dried apricots
Dried figs
Eggs
Haricot beans
Kidneys, liver
Meat
Mussels
Parsley
Peanuts
Peas
Red wine
Sardines
Shellfish
Spinach
Sprats
Sunflower seeds
Walnuts
Watercress
Wheatgerm | Anaemia
Loss of energy
Brittle nails
Premature grey nails
Breathlessness |

contd

Mineral	Food source	Function	Deficiency results in:	Daily need
Magnesium	Almonds Avocado pears Bran Brazil nuts Haricot beans Honey Meat Muesli Peanuts Seafood Wheatgerm Wholemeal cereals	Necessary for cell metabolism and nerve and muscle function	Muscular weakness Nervousness and depression Heart and circulatory diseases	300 mg
Phosphorous	Brewer's yeast Cheese Egg yolks Fish Liver Meat Wheatgerm	In combination with calcium, oxygen and hydrogen, forms the substance of bones. Play an important role in cell metabolism	Poor teeth and bones Disturbances in cell regulation	1000 mg
Potassium	Almonds Bananas Bran Brazil nuts Dried apricots Dried butter beans Figs Haricot beans Lentils Potatoes Soya beans Spinach Wheatgerm	Involved in the contraction of muscles, including that of the heart and in the transmission of nerve impulses. Helps regulate water balance. It is involved in female hormone activity; alleviates pre-menstrual tension	Muscular weakness Irritability	2500 mg

Mineral	Sources	Function	Deficiency symptoms	Recommended intake
Sodium	Bran Carrots Celery Dried pulses Lentils Meat Peas Salt Seafood Spinach Water	Associated with the contraction of muscles; transmission of nerve impulses in nerve fibres Maintenance of the electrolyte balance in the body	Protection against excess fluid loss (rare)	
Sulphur	Cheese Chicken Eggs Fish Haricot beans Meat Milk Nuts Soya beans	Essential for the formation of collagen which affects skin	Dry skin and hair Brittle nails (rare)	850 mg

Table 6.5 Minor minerals – trace elements

Mineral	Food source	Function	Deficiency results in:	Daily need
Chromium	Bran Brewer's yeast Chicken Fruit Green vegetables Honey Nuts Shellfish Wholegrain cereals	Assists in regulating blood sugar levels. May help to keep the cholesterol level down	Possible arteriosclerosis	Trace
Cobalt	Fruit Green vegetables Meat Wholegrain cereals	Necessary for function of vitamin B–12 and for erythrocytes	Anaemia Dry skin	Trace
Copper	Bran Brazil nuts Liver Shellfish Wheatgerm Wholegrain cereals	Together with iron in production of erythrocytes helps to form hair pigment	Grey hair Loss of hiar Anaemia (rare)	2–5 mg
Fluorine	Fish Seafood Tea Some drinking water	Counteracts tooth decay Helps to deposit calcium to strengthen bones and teeth	Tooth decay Soft bones and teeth	1 mg

Mineral	Sources	Functions	Deficiency	Amount
Iodine	Lettuce Seafood Sea salt Seaweed Shellfish Spinach	Necessary for the function of the thyroid hormones (thyroxine and triiodothyronine)	Dry skin Loss of hair	Trace
Manganese	Almonds Apricots Bran Kidneys Lentils Parsley Walnuts Watercress Wheatgerm	Influences blood sugar levels Helps to maintain reproductive processes	Lack of coordination Reduction in sexual activities Sterility (rare)	Trace
Zinc	Beans Bran Eggs Fish Onions Shellfish Sunflower seeds Wholewheat flour	Influences the enzyme and protein pattern in digestion	Retarded growth	Trace

If clients need a diet to reduce body weight it is important to enquire about their normal consumption of food. Find out if their diet has become imbalanced by eating too much carbohydrate in various forms (i.e. refined sugars and flours); also ensure that sufficient roughage or dietary fibre is being taken to provide bulk and satisfy the appetite. When they are only a few pounds overweight the cutting down of food is not always the answer. The real need is to balance the diet out correctly and increase daily exercise. A well-balanced diet with an increase in proteins is required for those clients wishing to put on body weight.

A poor diet can affect weight, complexion, strength and general well-being. Therefore, advise a variety of foods at each meal so that the body receives all the vitamins and minerals required without the need for supplements, i.e. vitamin pills.

Obesity

An increase of body weight by 10 per cent or more above the weight expected by the client's height and frame is considered as obesity. Although people vary in their tendency to put on fat, obesity is usually the result of eating more than the body requires, i.e. when the intake of food exceeds the energy needs of the body. Apart from being unattractive, too many extra pounds are a strain on the body and can also shorten the span of life. The overweight person is inviting a number of unnecessary complications, i.e. shortness of breath, high blood pressure, heart attack, diabetes mellitus and arteriosclerosis (hardening of the arteries, which is the result of fibrous and mineral deposits in the middle layer of the artery wall), or atherosclerosis (where fatty substances collect in the inner lining of the arteries to form plaques), apart from chronic back and joint pain due to the increased strain on joints and ligaments.

Some overweight people delude themselves into thinking that their extra pounds are caused by glandular disturbances, but this is rarely the case and can always be checked by the client's doctor. There could be hidden factors encouraging the overweight, i.e. drugs, etc., but these do not result in obesity.

The most important factor in losing weight is the determination to do so and the will to remain at the reduced weight when this is achieved. The beauty therapist can advise on diet, give a suitable exercise routine and suggest certain body treatments in the salon to help motivate the client to lose weight.

Anorexia nervosa

This is commonly known as the 'slimmer's disease' because it happens when a person starts dieting to become slim and allows it to go too far. However, its cause is far more complex than any simple desire to lose weight. Anorexia nervosa usually strikes young people between the ages of 11 and 30 and affects more females than males. The underlying cause is usually anxiety in some form or another, i.e. lack of confidence, a feeling of inadequacy or even the inability to progress from adolescence to maturity, so the cure is not simply weight gain. It is an illness which requires a complete change of mental outlook by the anorexic and considerable understanding by those in close contact. The obvious physical signs of anorexia nervosa are the dramatic weight loss, very thin limbs with bones protruding and an increase in body hair.

The beauty therapist will not see all the behavioural signs, for example, the smuggling away of food, the pretence of eating food, food binges followed by vomiting and the undue interest in laxatives, all of which the anorexic will believe are in the interest of being slim, but never thin! Medical help should be sought long before symptoms are acute. Unfortunately the beauty therapist is rarely able to assist before medical treatment has been given as the anorexic is usually anti-social and withdrawn and seldom visits the salon. Once a female client is on the road to recovery, treatments can be given in the salon to enhance her appearance, i.e. skin care and make-up lessons, to give her more self-confidence.

Bulimia

Bulimia and anorexia nervosa are the two extreme poles of the same world. Bulimic people have a morbid fear of gaining weight and yet they can have an irresistible urge to eat – without appetite or pleasure – as fast as possible and in great quantities. This is followed by humiliation, the feeling of failure and depression and, of course, the inevitable cycle of vomiting/purging/fasting before eating again. In the salon it will be very difficult to be aware of the bulimic client and therefore the beauty therapist can rarely help.

The digestive system

The digestive system performs the task of converting the food we eat into nutrients to nourish all the cells of the body It consists of the *alimentary canal* (or digestive tract) and adjoining *accessory organs* and together they compose the system whereby complex changes occur in ingested food materials. This happens by:

● *ingestion*, the taking of food into the alimentary canal,
● *digestion*, the breaking down of food substances physically by mastication (chewing) and also by splitting them chemically into simpler compounds by *enzymes* present in secretions produced by glands and accessory organs (an enzyme is a substance, usually protein in nature, that initiates and accelerates a chemical reaction in other substances while remaining unchanged in the process); the secretions produced are:
  ● saliva, from the salivary glands,
  ● gastric juice, from the stomach,
  ● pancreatic juice, from the pancreas,
  ● bile, from the liver,
  ● intestinal juice, from the small intestine.

● *absorption* is the process whereby food substances, which are digested, pass through the walls of some of the organs of the alimentary canal into the blood and lymph capillaries.
● *elimination* is the expulsion of waste material from the body.

The alimentary canal itself is a long passage (over 30 ft or 9 m) commencing at the mouth and terminating at the anus and consists of the mouth, the pharynx, the oesophagus, the stomach, the small intestine, the large intestine, the rectum and anal canal (see Fig. 6.1).

The accessory organs consist of the salivary glands, pancreas, liver and the biliary tract.

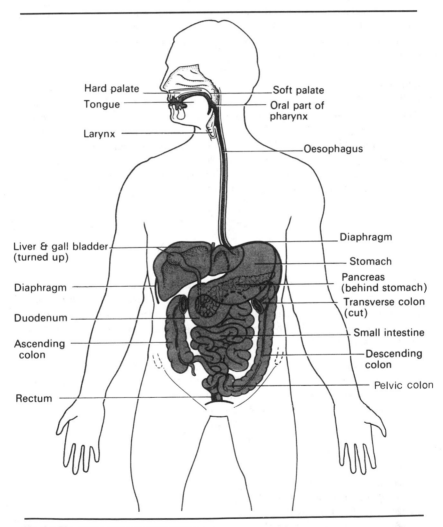

Fig. 6.1 The organs of the digestive system

The mouth

The mouth (or oral cavity) forms the beginning of the digestive system whereby chewing (or mastication) of the food takes place. It is also the site of the organs of taste, tongue (see *Special senses*, Chap. 3) and the lips and teeth. Except for the teeth, the mouth is lined with a mucous membrane. The *palate* forms the roof of the mouth: the front two-thirds comprise the *hard* palate (which is supported by the maxilla and the palatine bones) and the third at the back is the *soft* palate (which is hinged to the hard palate with the tonsils lying on either side). In the middle of the soft palate is the uvula which points down to the tongue and at the root of the tongue, below the uvula, lies the epiglottis. The tongue plays an important part in mastication and deglutition (swallowing).

The 32 permanent teeth in the adult are equally divided between the upper and lower jaw and are embedded in the sockets of the alveolar ridges of the mandible and maxilla. The ridges are bone which is covered by mucus membrane forming the gums (see Fig. 6.2). Teeth have varying shapes as they have different functions. They are arranged (in both upper and lower jaw) as follows:

- incisors 4,
- canine 2,
- premolars 4,
- molars 6.

The incisors (chisel shaped) and the canine (pointed crown) are the teeth used for cutting and biting food, whereas the premolars (two projections)

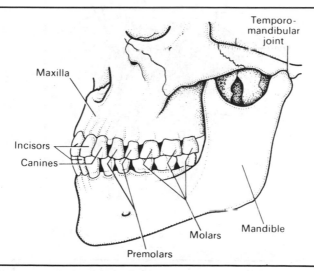

Fig. 6.2 The permanent teeth and the jaw bones

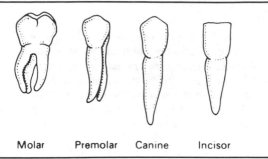

Molar   Premolar   Canine   Incisor

Fig. 6.3 The shapes of the permanent teeth

and molars (four or five projections) are used for grinding or chewing food. See Fig. 6.3 for the shapes of permanent teeth.

Each tooth is made up of three parts, the crown, the root and the neck. The crown is the part that protrudes from the gum, the root is the part which looks like fangs embedded in the alveolar processes of the jaw bones and the neck is the slightly constricted part which joins the crown with the root. In the centre of each tooth is the pulp cavity containing the nerve endings and blood vessels which nourish the tooth. This is covered by a hard, bony

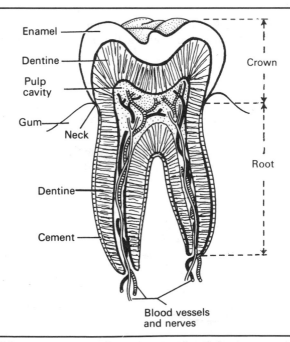

Fig. 6.4 A section of a tooth

substance called *dentine* and the dentine in the crown is covered by a thin layer of even harder substance, the *enamel*. The root of the tooth is covered with a bone-like substance called *cement* and this fixes the tooth in its socket (see Fig. 6.4).

The salivary glands

There are three pairs of glands which pour their secretions into the mouth through their ducts and these are:

- 2 parotid, one on each side of the face;
- 2 submandibular, which lie under the angle of the jaw, on either side of the face; and
- 2 sublingual, which lie under the mucous membrane of the floor of the mouth (see Fig. 6.5).

Saliva is the combined secretions from these glands. It consists of water, mineral elements, mucus and an enzyme called *salivary amylase* which converts cooked starch into maltose and dextrose. When food has been masticated by the teeth and moved around the mouth by the tongue and muscles of the cheeks, saliva softens and lubricates the food, so forming a soft mass or *bolus* ready for deglutition. Saliva also moistens the inside of the mouth, the tongue and the teeth and finally rinses them after the food has departed on the next stage of its journey.

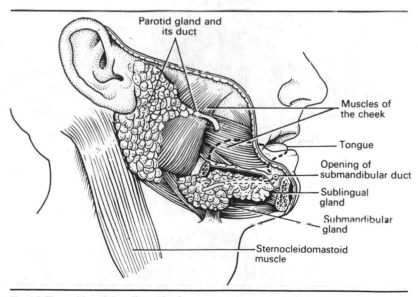

Fig. 6.5 The position of the salivary glands

The pharynx

This has been described in Chapter 5 whereby the nasal pharynx is separated from the mouth by the soft palate and uvula which close the nasal passages during deglutition while the epiglottis blocks off the larynx to allow food to pass into the oesophagus and not into the lower respiratory tract.

The oesophagus

The oesophagus, a muscular tube about 10 in (25 cm) long, is continuous with the pharynx above and lies in front of the vertebral column, behind the trachea and the heart. It passes through the diaphragm where it curves upwards to join the stomach (see Fig. 6.6). *Peristalsis*, i.e. waves of muscular

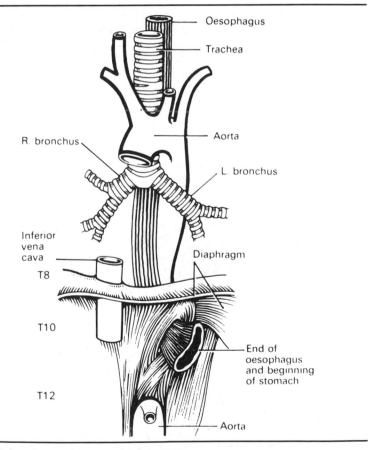

Fig. 6.6 Oesophagus and some associated structures

contraction, occurs to propel the bolus through the oesophagus and through the *cardiac orifice* (or sphincter) to the stomach.

The stomach

The stomach is a curved, muscular, sac-like structure which is continuous with the oesophagus at the cardiac orifice and at its lower end leads by way of the *pyloric orifice* to the duodenum, i.e. the proximal portion of the small intestine (see Fig. 6.7).

The walls of the stomach consist of four coats:

- an outer serous coat, the *peritoneum*, which has two layers; the parietal layer lines the abdominal wall and the visceral layer covers the organs in the abdomen and pelvis;
- a muscular coat, which is made up of circular, longitudinal and oblique muscle fibres;
- a sub-mucous coat which consists of loose connective tissue; and
- a mucous coat or membrane forming the inner lining.

Digestive juices (gastric juice) and mucus are added to the food in the stomach from the glands in this lining.

Gastric juice contains the enzymes pepsin and lipase. Pepsin breaks down proteins and converts them into peptones and also has a milk-clotting action similar to that of rennin and therefore facilitates the digestion of milk protein.

Lipase catalyses the decomposition of fats into glycerin and fatty acids. It is

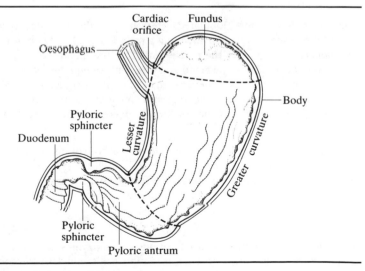

Fig. 6.7 Longitudinal section of the stomach

a rather weak fat-splitting enzyme in the stomach as it is only able to act on fats emulsified already, such as those in cream or the yolk of an egg. The *intrinsic factor*, a protein compound, found in the juice, is necessary for the absorption of vitamin B12 contained in food which is essential for the production of the anti-anaemia factor. The juice also contains *mucin* which coats and protects the stomach lining from becoming damaged by acid. *Hydrochloric acid* helps to dissolve the food and kills bacteria, but it also stops salivary amylase working as this enzyme cannot function in acidic surroundings. The amount of digestive juices is governed both here and in the intestine by nerve impulses, the presence of food itself and the secretion of hormones. The hormone *gastrin* stimulates the stomach cells to release hydrochloric acid and pepsin, once the food is in the stomach, but stops its secretion when the acidity reaches a certain point.

Food and drink enter the stomach relatively quickly and the stomach muscles contract in rhythm and gently churn these to a semi-fluid, partially digested mass, called *chyme* which is released through the pyloric sphincter into the duodenum, where pancreatic juice and bile enter the digestive tract.

The stomach reaches its peak of digestive activity approximately 2–3 hours after a meal but this will depend on the size of the meal and the type of food eaten. Carbohydrates leave the stomach more quickly than proteins and proteins more rapidly than fats

Care should be given to advise good eating habits to prevent stomach disturbances, i.e. indigestion and nausea. Two common forms of gastric discomfort are belching, which is usually associated with swallowing air while eating, and heartburn which is often caused by eating food too quickly.

The pancreas

The pancreas is a soft, lobulated, greyish-pink gland located below and behind the stomach and the liver. It has a rounded head, long body and a tail. The *pancreatic duct* runs the entire length of the gland, receiving smaller ducts from the lobules of the gland and joins the *common bile duct* as it opens into the duodenum to form the *ampulla of the bile duct* (see Fig. 6.8).

The pancreas is both an endocrine and an exocrine organ. The endocrine portion of the pancreas is the *islets of Langerhans* and these secrete two hormones:

- *insulin*, which plays a major role in carbohydrate metabolism and reduces the level of glucose in the blood; and
- *glucagon*, which has the opposite effect to that of insulin, increases the level of glucose in the blood particularly between meals when it is being used up during metabolism.

The main bulk of the gland is exocrine and is composed of cells that produce *pancreatic juice* containing a variety of digestive enzymes, i.e. mainly trypsinogen for breaking down proteins to amino acids, amylase for converting starch to maltose, and lipase for changing emulsified oils to glycerin and fatty

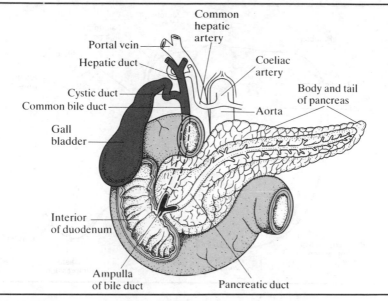

Fig. 6.8 The pancreas in relation to the duodenum and biliary tract. Part of the anterior wall of the duodenum removed

acids. The secretion of the juice is stimulated by the hormone *secretin*, which is produced by the duodenum lining when acid chyme enters from the stomach.

The liver

The liver is the largest gland in the body, red in colour and located in the upper right region of the abdomen, just below the diaphragm. It is divided into four lobes; the right lobe which is the largest, the left lobe which is wedge-shaped and smaller, and two lobes on the posterior surface, namely caudate and quadrate (see Fig. 6.9). The lobes of the liver are made up of masses of small lobules which are flat-sided and fit against each other and are encircled by small veins and arteries.

Within the lobules, branches of the portal vein and hepatic artery deliver nutrients and oxygenated blood to the *sinusoids* (little reservoirs surrounding the rows of liver cells – hepatocytes). These absorb and process nutrients and waste. Processed substances are returned to the sinusoids and leave via the intralobular vein (see Fig. 6.10). Waste, however, does not return to the bloodstream but leaves in the bile canaliculi (i.e. small channels running between the columns of hepatocytes) until they join up and eventually form the right and left hepatic ducts which drain bile from the liver.

Bile is a clear yellow or orange fluid produced by the liver. It is concentrated and stored in the gall bladder until it is needed for digestion. Bile salts

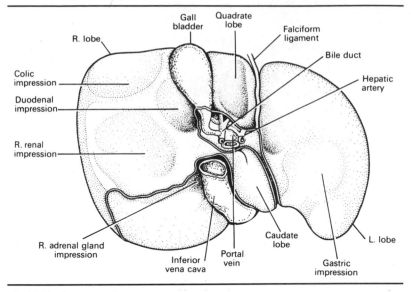

Fig. 6.9 The liver – posterior view

emulsify fats by breaking up large fat globules into smaller ones so that they can be acted on by the fat-splitting enzymes of the intestine and pancreas.

The main functions of the liver are to:

store glycogen from glucose by the action of insulin and convert glycogen to glucose by the action of adrenalin and glucagon to provide chemical energy;

desaturate fats into fatty acids and glycerol for storage and metabolism;

convert to glucose some amino acids produced from metabolism of protein; unwanted amino acids are deaminated and converted into urea and uric acid which are waste products discharged into the blood and excreted by the kidneys;

● produce heat;

store iron, and fat-soluble vitamins (A, D, K,) and B12;

manufacture some of the proteins of blood plasma and most of the blood-clotting factors from the available amino acids;

detoxicate poisons from the blood;

secrete bile.

The biliary tract

Bile ducts
There are three canals or passageways that conduct bile:

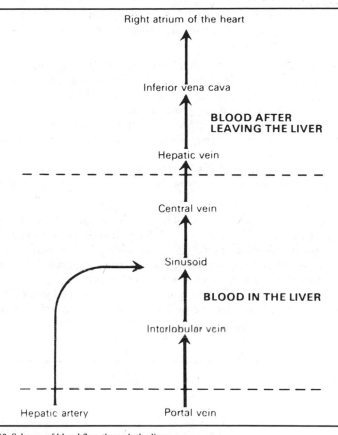

Right atrium of the heart

Inferior vena cava

**BLOOD AFTER
LEAVING THE LIVER**

Hepatic vein

Central vein

Sinusoid

BLOOD IN THE LIVER

Interlobular vein

Hepatic artery   Portal vein

Fig. 6.10 Scheme of blood flow through the liver

- the hepatic ducts which drain bile from the liver;
- the cystic duct (an extension of the gall bladder) which conveys bile from the gall bladder; and
- the common bile duct which passes through the wall of the small intestine at the duodenum and joins with the pancreatic duct (see Fig. 6.8).

The gall bladder
This is a small sac-like organ located below the liver and its main function is to act as a storage place for bile. It also absorbs water (so concentrating the bile) and its membrane adds mucus to the bile.

The small intestine
The digestive process continues in the small intestine which is a convoluted

tube about 20 ft (5 m) long. It extends from the stomach at the pyloric orifice and leads into the large intestine at the *ileocaecal valve.*

It consists of three parts:

● the *duodenum*, which is a C-shaped curve about 10 in (25 cm) long, and is the first and widest part of the small intestine; Note in Fig. 6.11 the head of the pancreas lies in this curve; the pancreatic juice, with its enzymes that break down starch, proteins and fats, flows into the duodenum together with the contents of the common bile duct (see Fig. 6.11);
● the *jejunum*, the middle part of the small intestine, which is about 7 ft (2 m) long; and
● the *ileum*, the terminal and narrowest section of the small intestine, which is about 10 ft (3 ms) long and ends at the ileocaecal valve (see Fig. 6.12).

The structure of the walls of the small intestine is similar to the stomach walls except that the formation of the internal lining is different. It has deep folds and finger-like projections called *villi* which assist in the absorption of food and contain tiny blood and lymphatic vessels and small glands. These glands secrete the *intestinal juice* (namely succus entericus) containing water, mucus and the enzymes sucrose, maltose and lactose, protease and lipase. It is this juice which completes the digestion whereby carbohydrates, proteins and fats are broken down into sugars, amino acids, fatty acids and glycerin. Absorp-

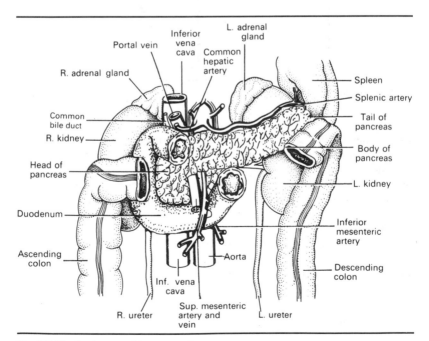

Fig. 6.11 The duodenum and its associated structures

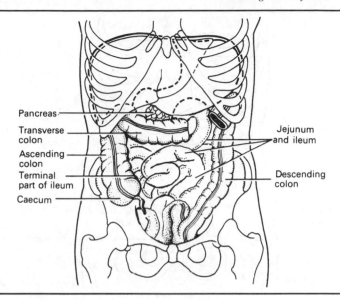

Fig. 6.12 The jejunum and ileum and their associated structures

tion of the products of digestion is completed in the small intestine. Any indigestible parts of food pass into the large intestine.

The large intestine, rectum and anal canal

The large intestine (or colon)
This is about 5 ft (1.5 m) in length and, as will be seen in Fig. 6.13, it almost surrounds the small intestine. It is divided into:

- the *caecum*, which is the first part of the colon; it consists of a lined pouch, from which extends a small blind tube, namely the *vermiform appendix* (see Fig. 6.13); the remainder of undigested food, roughage (cellulose) and unabsorbed digestive juices pass into the caecum as fluid;
- the *ascending colon* passes upward from the caecum to the lower edge of the liver, where it bends and becomes
- the *transverse colon*; this part of the colon lies across the abdominal cavity from right to left (below the stomach), and then bends downwards to become
- the *descending colon*; this part of the colon extends downwards along the left side of the abdomen; when it enters the pelvis it is known as
- the *pelvic colon* (sigmoid flexure), which is an S-shaped curve extending down to the sacrum where it becomes the rectum.

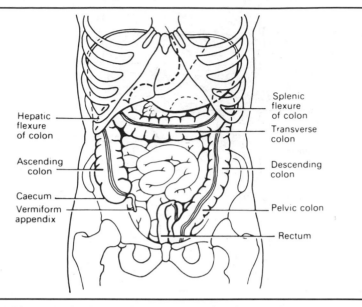

Fig. 6.13 Diagram showing the parts of the large intestine (colon) and their positions

The rectum

This is a slightly dilated part of the colon between the pelvic colon and the anal canal.

The anal canal

This leads from the rectum to the exterior. This canal has two circular (sphincter) muscles, internal and external, which control the anus, allowing the evacuation of faeces.

Water and some mineral salts are absorbed in the large intestine through the intestinal walls and so waste is formed into fairly solid faeces and pushed down into the rectum for eventual elimination. There are large numbers of microbes present in the colon and in the faeces but these do not normally cause disease.

Metabolism

In general terms, metabolism refers to all the chemical processes occurring within our bodies that allow growth, survival and reproduction. Essentially these processes are concerned with the disposition of the nutrients absorbed into the blood following digestion.

Metabolism is the product of two quite distinct and complementary processes, namely:

- *catabolism*, which consists of the breakdown of carbohydrates, proteins and fats to provide energy and a number of waste products; the energy released by catabolism is converted into useful work through muscle activity and a certain amount is lost as heat; and
- *anabolism*, which is concerned with the constructive processes by which nutrients are adapted to be stored as energy or used by the body in growth, e.g. by building up of muscle from amino acids, reproduction and defence against infections.

The energy produced in the body may be measured and expressed in units of work (*kilojoules*) or units of heat (*calories*). One calorie is the amount of heat required to raise the temperature of 1 litre of water through 1 degree (1°) Celsius (C). (This is about the same as the amount of heat required to raise the temperature of 1 lb of water by 4° Fahrenheit.) It is possible to calculate the amount of energy contained in certain food by measuring the amount of heat units, or calories, in that food. All energy content and output is measured in kilojoules, e.g. 1 calorie is equivalent to approximately 4.2 kilojoules. There are many books available detailing calorific values of foods.

The metabolic rate, i.e. the amount of energy a person burns up, has two components. One, the energy a person expends when he or she is completely at rest, which is called the basal metabolic rate, (BMR), and two, the amount of energy expended in muscular activity, which varies from BMR to something like 2,920 kJ/hour or 700 calories/hour for a person engaged in heavy work or strenuous sport.

Therefore, the amount of energy required for these chemical processes varies as factors such as weight, age, activity, etc. will determine the daily calorie requirement.

Metabolism of carbohydrates
When digested, carbohydrates are converted into simple sugars, i.e. glucose, fructose and galactose. These are first transported to the liver, where fructose and galactose are converted into glucose. In the liver, glucose can be used in several ways: some is used for energy and some becomes glycogen. Once the glycogen storage areas are filled, the glucose is converted into fat, but can also be converted back to glucose if needed to meet extra energy requirements. The end-products of carbohydrate metabolism are energy, carbon dioxide and water.

Metabolism of protein
The end products of protein digestion, amino acids, pass into the blood, some to be used as structural proteins for the building of body tissues, others to be used as enzymes, and the rest to be carried to various parts of the body as a reserve. If a ready supply of carbohydrates is not available, some proteins may be converted into needed energy. Excess amino acids or those

unrequired for body-building are split up in the liver to form glucose for fuel and produce urea as a waste product.

Metabolism of fat

The products of fat digestion are absorbed through the intestinal walls and distributed by the blood to various storage regions in the body. The end-products of fat metabolism are energy, heat, carbon dioxide and water.

Chapter 7

The reproductive and urinary systems

The reproductive system

Reproduction is the process by which an organism produces a new individual. Both sexes produce specialised cells, called *gametes*, containing genetic material, namely *genes* and *chromosomes*. The gonads, ovaries in the female and testes in the male, produce the germ cells which are the male spermatozoon and the female ovum. Reproduction begins when the germ cells unite, a process called fertilisation.

The male reproductive systems consists of the external genitalia, accessory glands that secrete special fluids and the ducts through which these organs and glands are connected to each other and through which the spermatozoa are ejaculated during coitus. The knowledge of this system is not relevant to beauty therapy whereas the beauty therapist can give advice on the effects of female puberty, menstrual cycle, pregnancy, menopause and breast care pertaining to the female reproductive system.

The female reproductive system

The function of the female reproductive system is to form the ovum (egg) and, when it is fertilised, to carry the unborn child through to birth. The female reproductive organs, called *genitalia* lie in the bony pelvis and are divided into external and internal organs.

The external organs

These are collectively known as the *vulva* and comprise the following parts.

The mons pubis (or veneris) is the rounded fleshy prominence over the symphysis pubis. At puberty, this area becomes covered with hair.

The labia majora are the two thick folds which form the sides of the vulva and are composed of skin, fibrous tissue, sebaceous glands, blood vessels and nerves.

The labia minora (or nymphae)   are two small folds of skin between the labia majora and the opening of the vagina. Posteriorly they fuse to form the *fourchette* (see Fig. 7.1).

The clitoris   is a small, elongated, erectile body homologous with the penis in the male and is situated anteriorly in the vestibule.

The vestibule   is the space between the labia minora into which the urethra and vagina open. The *greater vestibular* (Bartholin's) *glands* lie just behind the labia majora, one on each side, and secrete mucus that keeps the vulva moist.

The hymen   is the membranous fold partly closing the vaginal orifice until it is ruptured either through the first sexual intercourse or more frequently through sports activities. Horse-riding, for example, is a common cause.

The perineum   in the pelvic floor is the region between the vaginal orifice and the anus which gives attachment to the muscles of the pelvic floor.

The internal organs

These consist of the following:

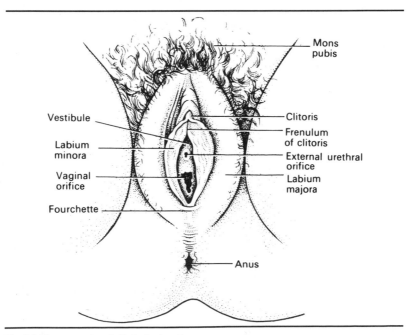

Fig. 7.1 The external genitalia in the female

The vagina is a muscular canal, lined with stratified epithelium and well supplied with blood vessels and nerves. It runs obliquely upwards and backwards from the vestibule to the uterus. The vagina is the passage for menstrual discharge and also stretches to many times its usual size during labour and childbirth.

The uterus, or womb is a hollow muscular organ lying in the female pelvic cavity between the urinary bladder and the rectum and is normally about the size and shape of a pear. The parts of the uterus are:

- *the fundus*, or upper part, which is broad and flattened;
- *the corpus*, or body, which is the middle portion;
- *the cervix*, the lower part, which is narrow and tubular.

The walls of the uterus are composed of three layers of tissue, perimetrium, myometrium and endometrium. The *perimetrium* consists of peritoneum, which is a serous membrane covering most of the surface of the uterus. The thickest layer of tissue in the uterine walls are composed of muscle fibres, namely, *myometrium* and the inner lining is called *endometrium* (see Fig. 7.2). Between puberty and the menopause, the lining goes through a monthly cycle of growth and discharge, known as the menstrual cycle.

The uterine tubes (or Fallopian tubes) are small slender tubes about 4 in (10 cm) long, extending laterally from the sides of the uterus, between the body and fundus. When the mature ovum leaves the ovary it enters the uterine tube through which it travels to the uterus. Fertilisation of the ovum usually takes place in the uterine tubes.

The ovaries are the gonads (sex glands) in the female. There are two

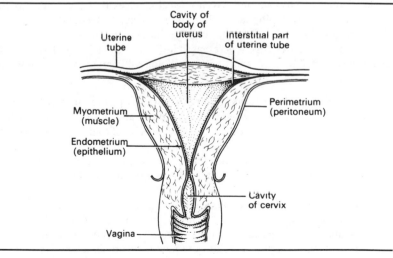

Fig. 7.2 Diagram of a section of the uterus

ovaries which are almond-shaped, usually the size of a large walnut, and each is attached by ligaments to the upper part of the uterus. Each ovary contains a large number of immature ova and at each menstrual cycle, one of these begins to mature and develop into a *Graafian* follicle.

As the follicle matures, it moves to the surface of the ovary and forms a projection. When fully matured, the Graafian follicle breaks open and releases the ovum which passes into the uterine tubes.

The release of the ovum is called *ovulation*. Maturation of the follicle is stimulated by a hormone from the anterior pituitary gland, namely the *FSH* (follicle stimulating hormone) and the lining cells of the follicle secretes *oestrogen*.

Once ovulation is complete the lining cells together with *LH* (the luteinizing hormone, also from the anterior pituitary gland) develop into a yellow body called the *corpus luteum* which secretes the hormone *progesterone*.

If the ovum is fertilised the corpus luteum continues to grow for several months to provide a good environment for the ovum to grow. If the ovum is not fertilised, the corpus luteum persists for only 12–14 days and then atrophies just before the onset of the next menstrual period.

Therefore the ovaries have two important functions, i.e. ovulation and the production of the two hormones, oestrogen and progesterone, which influence a woman's feminine characteristics and affect the process of reproduction (see Fig. 7.3).

Female puberty

Puberty is the stage of growth at which the reproductive organs reach maturity and in the female this varies between the ages of 10 and 14 years. There are a number of physical and psychological changes that take place as the body is usually developing faster than the mind can understand or the emotions control. Physically, there are changes in the appearance of the body as the vital hormone 'oestrogen' is released into the blood stream. The physical changes (external and internal) and psychological changes can be summarised as follows.

● *Externally*, the breasts will enlarge and develop; the vulva will enlarge and pubic hair will grow on the mons pubis and in the axillae; the face will become fuller; the body will become rounded to develop a waist and hips and there is an increase in the rate of growth. The sebaceous glands in the skin are activated and often, externally, teenage acne appears.
● *Internally*, oestrogen will be affecting changes in the body whereby the myometrium and endometrium will thicken, the uterus will enlarge and the menstrual cycle and ovulation will begin.
● *Psychologically*, the internal conflict of moving from childhood to womanhood creates uncertainty, physical appearance is changing but rarely quick enough to emulate the media advertisements. There is the loss of security as a child, but there is also the fear of independence as an

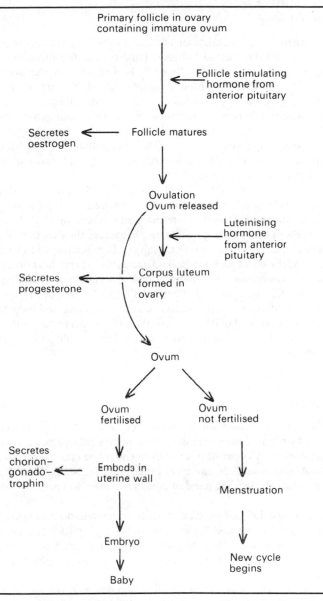

Fig. 7.3 A summary of the stages of development of the ovum and the associated hormones

adult which often results in moods and sometimes hostility. When young clients come into the salon, usually with skin problems, sympathy and understanding are as effective as the treatment given.

Menstrual cycle

The menstrual cycle consists of changes in the ovaries and uterine walls during a 26–30 day period between puberty and the menopause, except during pregnancy. This cycle of activity is controlled by the hypothalamus and operates through the anterior pituitary gland. During the first 9 or 10 days of the cycle the Graafian follicle matures, the endometrium is repaired and renewed and there is an increase in oestrogen resulting in ovulation. This is followed by a further 14 or so days where the corpus luteum produces progesterone. If the ovum is not fertilised menstruation occurs which usually lasts about 5 days when there is discharge from the vagina of blood and tissues from the non-pregnant uterus.

Due to the enormous hormonal changes which take place during each menstrual cycle, some women are subject to pre-menstrual tension (PMT), now more commonly known as pre-menstrual syndrome (PMS), resulting in a tenderness of the breasts, possible weight gain, or the experience of unpleasant mood changes. As a beauty therapist, there is little you can do except suggest that the client seek medical advice as there is medication available to relieve the symptoms. Alternative medical treatments, including homeopathic remedies, may also be effective in mitigating the symptoms of PMS. Homeopathy itself is a combination of natural healing and medical science but rejects the method of drug prescription. It is worth finding out if there is a practitioner in the surrounding area of the salon to enable advice to be given to the client.

Pregnancy

Usually the first indication of pregnancy is a missed menstrual period, followed by changes in the breasts as the nipples enlarge and the areola may become darker. A client who is pregnant should be encouraged to attend an antenatal clinic where she can meet other pregnant women and experienced teachers who can clear the mind of doubts and fears and prepare the body for birth.

There are specially adapted exercises for women to do during pregnancy to keep the body strong and flexible and to get back into shape more quickly after the baby is born. Posture and breathing are very important and need special attention and a beauty therapist can advise certain exercises (see Chapter 8).

Advice can also be given on nutrition and diet as it is important to avoid excess weight gain. Stretch marks are less likely to occur if the weight gain is kept to about 1/2 lb (249 gm) a week. Daily massage with olive oil or lanolin or even cocoa oil all over the abdomen and thighs may help to avoid these marks.

Regular oil manicures will help the nails as these can prove difficult during pregnancy. Skin is twice as active, which means it can improve more quickly, and usually requires frequent cleansing. Skin traditionally looks better due to the fact that pregnancy raises the oestrogen level in the body. Pigmentation marks sometimes appear but these vanish when the baby is born.

Menopause

Menopause occurs when changes take place in the ovaries and ovulation and the menstrual cycles become irregular and gradually stop. This usually takes place between the ages of 45 and 55 years. It may occur quite suddenly or over a period of several years. Physiological changes occur because the oestrogen secretion stops and these include atrophy of the sex organs, shrinkage of the breasts and a thinning of the axillary and pubic hair. Most women pass through the menopause with little discomfort. However, there are some symptoms which can be experienced and these include:

- a sensation of heat in the face and upper part of the body, namely, 'a hot flush' which can also be followed by sweating or palpitations;
- fatigue or sudden spells of weeping;
- inability to concentrate or poor memory; and
- insomnia.

A very few women may have a more severe reaction resulting in depression. All these symptoms are treated by the medical profession but as a beauty therapist you can help in some areas. It must be remembered that the menopause happens at a time when a woman becomes aware of ageing, children leaving home, the loss of older relatives and the feeling of not being wanted or needed. With all the years spent helping others, the beauty therapist can help the client improve her self-awareness, on a physical level at least, particularly by encouraging an improvement in her figure and skin.

Breasts (or mammary glands)

In women the breasts are the secondary sex organs and their main function is to produce milk after childbirth. In the male they neither function nor develop. The breasts lie over the pectoral muscles and are supported by the suspensory ligaments of Cooper (see Chapter 2). The two ovarian hormones, oestrogen and progesterone, control their development during puberty. Oestrogen stimulates growth of the ducts of the mammary glands and the progesterone stimulates development of the alveoli.

Breast size is mainly determined by the amount of fat around the glandular tissue rather than the amount of glandular tissue itself. Connective tissue covers the glandular tissue which in turn is sheathed in a layer of fatty tissue. It is the fatty tissue which gives the breast its smooth outline and acts as a significant factor in its size and firmness.

Each breast consists of approximately 20 lobes and each lobe consists of several lobules. These are composed of connective tissue in which are embedded the secreting cells, i.e. alveoli of the gland which open into small ducts. These ducts unite to form *lactiferous ducts* and along their length, the ducts have widened areas that form reservoirs in which milk can be stored and these are called *lactiferous sinuses*. The ducts then narrow to pass through the nipple and open on to its surface. The nipple itself consists of skin and erectile tissue, dark in colour, and it is perforated by 15 to 20 orifices which are the milk ducts of the gland. The nipple is surrounded by an area called the *areola* (see Fig. 7.4).

Breast care

The most common cancers in women are those of the breasts, the cervix and uterus, but it is breast cancer that women fear most. Women should examine their breasts on a regular monthly basis as early detection of any irregularities or lumps has a far better chance of being successfully treated. It is important that you advise a client that if a lump is found, however small, immediate medical advice should be sought. At the same time, it is equally important that you allay the fear the client will have, as fear often delays a visit to the doctor. Statistics indicate that 65–80 per cent of all breast lumps are not cancerous but are benign nodules, containing liquid, which have no malignant potential.

Quite often clients will ask how they can make a self-examination of their breasts, especially if they are embarrassed to seek medical advice. The best time for this is just after menstruation when the breasts are normally soft and at their smallest or, for women past the menopause, at monthly intervals.

Advise the client to:

● stand in front of a mirror with arms at the sides and note if there is any

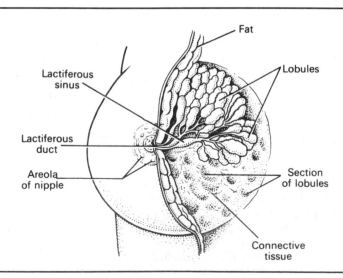

Fig. 7.4 The breast

dimpling, change in the shape of the breast or any change in the nipples;
look for any sign of bleeding or unusual discharge;

raise the arms above the head and check again for similar symptoms;

lie on the bed and put a small towel under one shoulder to help spread
the breast tissue; with one arm under the head, imagine the breast as
being divided into four quarters of a circle;

place the free hand, with the four fingers together; gently but firmly
begin by examining the inner upper quarter; start feeling well out from
the breast and work towards the nipple;

in the same way, examine the inner lower quarter, i.e. starting from the
breast bone and from the ribs below the breast towards the nipple;

bring the arm down to the side and start to feel the outer, lower quarter,
i.e. from the ribs below and at the side of the breast and work towards
the nipple;

feel the upper quarter until you have completed the circle;

finally, feel for any lumps in the armpit and examine the nipple itself by
pressing gently, again feeling for any lumps.

The same sequence should be followed for the other breast. The appearance
of any of these symptoms may be insignificant, but the client should be
advised to see her own doctor as soon as possible.

The urinary system

The urinary system consists of those organs that produce urine and eliminate
it from the body and is formed by the kidneys, ureters, urinary bladder and
the urethra (see Fig. 7.5 for parts of this system).

The kidneys

There are two kidneys and these lie on the posterior abdominal wall, on
either side of the vertebral column (see Fig. 7.6). They are bean-shaped
organs, about 4 in (11 cm) long, 2 in (6 cm) wide and 1 in (3 cm) thick, and a
heavy cushion of fat normally encases each kidney and holds it in place.

The kidney consists of an outer part called the *cortex* and an inner part
called the *medulla*. Each kidney contains over a million microscopic filtering
units called *nephrons*.

The nephron resembles a tiny funnel with a very long stem, parts of which
are highly convoluted. It is closed at one end and at the other end it opens
into a *collecting tubule*.

As will be seen in Fig. 7.7 the closed end is indented to form the *glomerular
capsule* or *Bowman's capsule*, which encloses the *glomerulus* (a network of
arterial capillaries which is supplied with blood by an afferent arteriole with
branches from the renal artery). The remainder of the nephron is divided in
three parts:

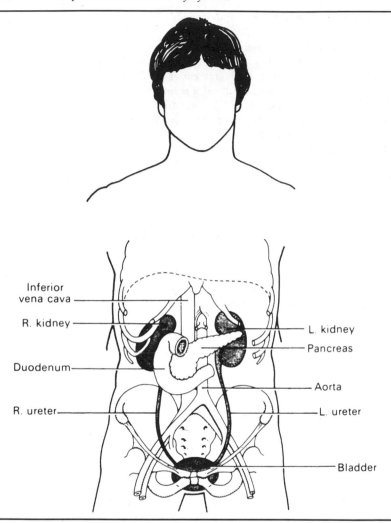

Fig. 7.5 The parts of the urinary system and some associated structures

- the *proximal convoluted tubule*, nearest to the Bowman's capsule;
- the *loop of Henle*, a U-shaped portion of the nephron between the proximal and distal convoluted portions; and
- the *distal convoluted tubule*, located distally to the Bowman's capsule, leading into a collecting tubule.

The capsules and convoluted tubules lie in the cortex, and the loop of Henle and collecting tubules in the medulla. Urine is formed by means of two processes, ultra-filtration and selective reabsorption.

Ultra-filtration   is the first step in urine formation. It is a process whereby the high pressure of the blood that passes through the glomerulus forces water, glucose, urea and salts through the capillary walls to be collected by the Bowman's capsule.

Selective reabsorption from the nephron tubules into the blood capillaries surrounding the tubules is the second step in urine formation. The filtrate collected by the Bowman's capsule passes into the proximal convoluted tubule, where glucose, some salts and some water are absorbed. It then passes through the loop of Henle, the major site of water reabsorption and through the distal convoluted tubule where salt and water are absorbed. Normally all the glucose is reabsorbed, but in diabetics some occurs in the urine.

Excess water and other waste materials remain in the tubules as urine. Urine contains, besides water, a quantity of urea, uric acid, yellow pigments from the breakdown of haemoglobin, and salts, and moves through the ureters to the bladder for excretion.

The amount of urine is:

● *increased* by high water intake, emotional stress or nervousness, or diuretics, e.g. caffeine;
● *decreased* by high salt intake and by conditions which result in sweating, e.g. fevers and exercise.

Functions of the kidneys are:

● to maintain the normal acid balance of the body;

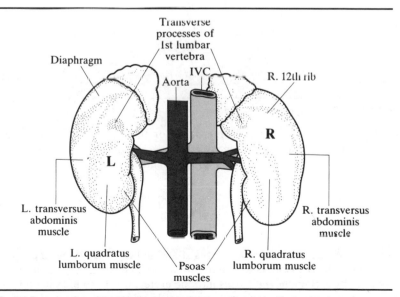

Fig. 7.6 Posterior view of the kidneys showing the areas of contact with associated structures

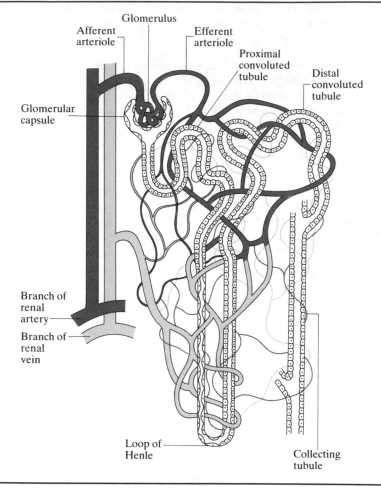

Fig. 7.7 Diagram of a nephron including the arrangement of the blood vessels

- to maintain the chemical composition of the fluids in the body, i.e. amounts of sodium and potassium;
- to excrete the end products of protein metabolism, e.g. urea and uric acid;
- to excrete certain drugs.

The ureters

The ureters are narrow muscular tubes, 10–12 in (25–30 cm) long, that conduct urine from the kidneys to the urinary bladder (see Fig. 7.8). As urine is produced by each kidney, it passes into the ureter, which, contracting rhythmically, forces the urine along and empties it in spurts into the bladder.

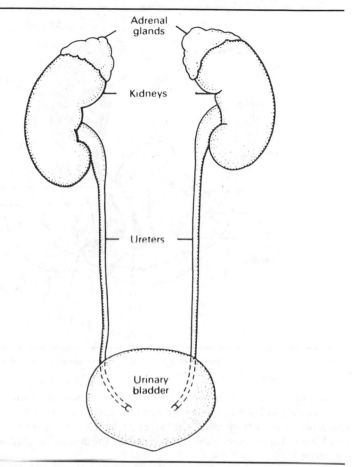

Fig. 7.8 The ureters and their relationships to the kidneys and bladder

The urinary bladder

The urinary bladder is a hollow container with muscular walls acting as a reservoir for urine. It is joined to the kidneys by ureters and to the exterior of the body by the urethra. Urine passes to the bladder from the kidneys every few seconds and remains there until it is emptied. Micturition occurs when the sphincters at the juncture of the bladder and urethra are relaxed and the muscular walls of the bladder contract, forcing the urine out (see Fig. 7.9).

The urethra

The urethra is the canal extending from the bladder and opening to the outside of the body through which urine passes. Its length differs in the female and the male.

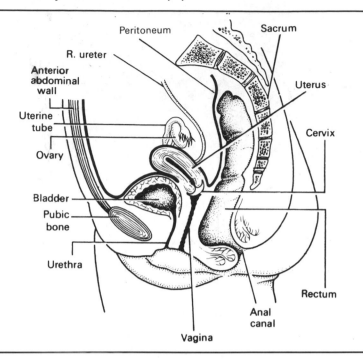

Fig. 7.9 The pelvic organs associated with the bladder and the urethra in the female

Cystitis is an inflammation of the bladder causing frequent and painful micturition with a burning sensation in the urethra. It is caused by bacterial infection usually from intestinal bacteria which are present in the anal area. In females these bacteria can easily enter the urethra unless careful hygiene is practised.

Chapter 8

Exercise

It is a well-known fact that our present society suffers most, in terms of health, from 'lifestyle-related problems'. One of the main reasons being the lack of physical activity in the work environment, especially with the advent of more sedentary occupations, such as those incorporating the use of computers. There are many misconceptions about fitness and exercise as it is often believed that exercise is only needed for sports activities and for the very young. A beauty therapist can give advice on a range of exercises to help improve the health and well-being of the individual. Exercise is vital to overall health as it promotes good circulation, increases oxygen intake, firms muscles and moves joints giving flexibility and suppleness. It can also help dispel nervous tensions, increase cardiac stamina, speed up the metabolic rate for the purpose of weight loss and delay some ageing symptoms.

Before giving any exercise programme the beauty therapist must have a sound knowledge of the skeletal and muscular systems and an understanding of how the body moves to be able to tailor the exercises for the individual's needs.

Mechanics of movement

Muscular contraction

There are three types of muscular contraction:

- *concentric* – where muscle shortens as it develops tension, i.e. when its origin and insertion move closer together;
- *eccentric* – where muscle lengthens as it develops tension; and;
- *static* – where muscle develops tension but retains its length, i.e. when its origin and insertion remain the same distance apart but the muscle thickens and becomes firm.

Range of muscle movement

- *Full range* is where a muscle works from full contraction to full stretch.

- *Middle range* is where the muscle is neither fully extended nor fully contracted.
- *Outer range* is where a muscle contracts from its furthest extent to its point of mid-contraction.
- *Inner range* is where a muscle contracts from its mid-point of contraction to its fullest point of contraction.

When exercising, shortened muscles should be worked eccentrically in the outer range and overstretched muscles should be worked concentrically in the inner range. Middle-range movement is the most commonly used and muscles are most efficient in this range.

Movement is brought about not just by one muscle contracting but by the interaction of different muscles performing different roles. This is known as the group action of muscles.

Group action of muscles

- *agonist* (or prime mover) is the muscle which brings about the required action normally contracting concentrically;
- *antagonist* relaxes allowing the required movement to take place;
- *synergist* contracts concentrically and assists the agonist in achieving the required movement; and
- *fixator* holds the joint or body part stable.

All muscle-work relies on an intact nervous system which receives and sends messages for the brain to interpret into patterns of movement.

Metabolism

When exercise is performed, the activity of the muscles requires an increase in their metabolism for the production of energy. This metabolism may be *aerobic* (using oxygen) or *anaerobic* (not using oxygen). Aerobic metabolism requires oxygen in increasing supplies which is brought to the active muscles by the blood. Therefore, the intensity of aerobic metabolism will be limited by the blood supply to the muscle. Energy is produced by the oxidation of foodstuffs, also transported by the blood. Glucose, lactic acid and fatty acids can be used by the body in this way. The waste products are carbon dioxide and water.

Breathing in exercise

In order to meet the increased oxygen requirements of exercising muscles, respiratory function undergoes a definite change during exercise. The volume of air breathed in during exercise is brought about by an increase in the rate and depth of breathing and these changes increase the work of the respiratory muscles, i.e. the diaphragm, intercostals and other accessory muscles of respiration. The resistance to air flow through the nose during breathing is higher than through the mouth, and so during active exercise respiration is usually switched from the nose to the mouth in order to attain the necessary volumes of air.

Above a certain level of activity it is possible that the delivery of oxygen cannot keep up with the energy demand and then energy must be produced anaerobically if activity is to continue. It is this process which leads to the condition known as *oxygen debt* and eventually to muscular fatigue. The oxygen debt is 'paid back' through deep breathing and prolonged increased circulation that occurs after the exercise is over.

When more vigorous exercise is performed, lactic acid is produced (by metabolism) so quickly that the mechanisms for oxidising it are overloaded. In any exercise it is important for the beauty therapist to watch the client's breathing, as breath held for a long period of time may cause intra-thoracic pressure which decreases circulation to the brain and fainting may result.

Fatigue

Fatigue usually occurs in two ways, i.e.

● if blood flow through the muscle is inadequate to remove the lactic acid formed, the latter will accumulate in the muscle and inhibit further contraction;
● anaerobic processes may cause muscular fatigue by exhaustion of the stores of glycogen (glucose) in the muscle but this is rare.

Fatigue caused by increasing lactic acid concentration is usually alleviated within the hour.

Fitness tests

It is important that each client exercises to his/her own level of fitness, which depends on the individual's general state of health. One test is to measure the pulse recovery rate and this should be done before taking any exercise and then *immediately* after ceasing a particular part of the exercise programme, as the pulse rate will decrease rapidly even within the first minute after exercise.

In taking the pulse, place three fingers over the radial artery (or under the mandible in the side of the neck) and it should be possible to feel the pulsations as the heart pumps. The pulse rate can be timed for 20 seconds and then multiplied by three to give heart beats per minute (see Chapter 4). It is necessary for all clients to be able to take their own pulse rate, and time spent on this part of the programme at the beginning of a course is time well spent.

Again dependent on the fitness of each client it may be necessary to introduce an 'unfitness handicap'. For those who have not exercised for a long time, are obese or who smoke, an initial handicap of 40 would be advisable but this can always be re-assessed as fitness improves. The figure of 200, minus the age of the client, minus 40 for unfitness indicates the upper safety level of heart beats per minute, i.e. HBM. eg:

```
   200
 −  40 years of age
 −  40 unfitness handicap
 =120 HBM
```

Post exercise pulse rates should be checked to determine that they fall within safe levels but if these are exceeded then a period of rest is recommended until the pulse rate comes down before continuing with light exercise.

Area, equipment, clothing and footwear

Area   for an individual client all that is required is sufficient floor space on which to lie and room in which to turn around without obstruction, when the arms are fully extended. Therefore, the area of floor space is determined by the number of clients participating in an exercise class. Ensure that the floor area is anti-slip to avoid accidents and that the room is well-ventilated.

Equipment   initially can be very minimal. e.g. towels or blankets on which to lie (this can be extended to yoga mats). Small types of gymnastic equipment, such as hoops and rings and small hand weights, will help to vary the exercise programme. For an established class more sophisticated equipment can be purchased, i.e. static bicycles, rowing machines and general weight-training machines. For safety reasons all apparatus should be checked regularly for wear and tear.

Clothing   should be comfortable, supportive but not restrictive, i.e. loose tops and shorts, leotards, bathing suits, underwear, etc. Women, especially those with large breasts, should wear a bra that has enough stretch in it to allow movement but prevents the breasts from wobbling up and down. There are bras available that have no fastenings, trimmings or bindings (which can chafe) and have a broad band under the bust (this ensures that the bra does not ride up).

Footwear   is dependent on the type of exercise undertaken and can vary from bare-feet to ballet-type slippers to training shoes. If the exercise class combines jogging, jumping and twisting, a suitable training or sports shoe should be advised. The shoe should have a high top to support the ankles and a dip at the back for the achilles tendon, with cushioning at the ball and heel of the shoe to absorb small shocks of impact and avoid strained leg muscles or backache.

Contra-indications

These are very few as most exercises can be programmed to the client's ability. The figure diagnosis will alert the beauty therapist to any medical history and constant supervision will ensure that the client remains within his/her capabilities without over-exertion. On occasions where figure diagnosis is not possible the therapist should advise clients to seek medical advice if:

there is a history of high blood pressure or heart disease;
they have pains in their joints or back, or if they have arthritis;
they have any chest problems, i.e. asthma or bronchitis;
they have sugar diabetes;
● they are recovering from an operation.

Medical checks should also by taken by clients over 30 years of age who are contemplating a vigorous exercise routine.

Exercises should not be given within two hours of eating a heavy meal or while under the influence of alcohol

Planning an exercise programme

Having assessed the condition, occupation, sex and age of the client, take pulse rates while resting and again after two minutes of exercise.

If it is a general scheme, exercises for all parts of the body should be included and the first sessions should be fairly short and certainly not strenuous. The programme should include a balanced sequence of exercises, divided into mobility exercises for suppleness, exercises for strength and endurance exercises for stamina. i.e.

for suppleness, the maximum range of movements of the neck, spine and joints should be used to avoid straining ligaments and the pulling of muscles and tendons; the more mobile clients are, the less likely they are to suffer aches and pains brought on by stiffness;
for strength, which is the ability of muscles of the body to exert force (or torque) against a given resistance and therefore means extra muscle power for unexpected heavier work;
for stamina, which is the staying power, endurance, the ability to keep going without gasping for breath.

Basically, exercise is either static or dynamic, depending on whether or not it produces movement. In static exercises, called *isometrics*, muscles contract against resistance without any movement of the limbs. Although these are excellent exercises for building up muscles, they are not so good for increasing heart and lung efficiency and therefore they are not good enough on their own to promote fitness. In dynamic exercises, called *isotonic*, the limbs are moved rhythmically. The larger the muscles and the more vigorous the effort, the greater the demand for oxygen in the blood which improves vascular and respiratory circulation.

Breathing

Clients should be taken through breathing exercises and a simple one to follow is as follows.

Stand the client with the feet slightly apart and the hands on the lower part of the ribs with the fingertips just touching. As the client breathes in, the ribs will rise and expand, so pushing the fingers apart, and as the client exhales slowly, the ribs will close inwards and the fingers will touch again. Clients should be encouraged to breathe deeply to improve their respiration.

Warm-up exercises

Always commence a class with suitable 'warm-up' exercises which should be gradual and reasonably gentle to increase general circulation (warm-up muscles and loosen joints) and so reduce the likelihood of strain.

● Start with a *super-stretch*, standing with legs about 9 ins (23 cm) apart and with arms above the head. Use the arms to imitate climbing an imaginary rope ensuring a good stretch for each 'climb' (see Fig. 8.1).
● *Hand circling* will exercise the shoulders and upper arms. Standing with feet apart and arms out-stretched at shoulder level, small circles are made with the hands (see Fig. 8.2).
● *Firm the bust* by standing and folding the arms, i.e. grasping each forearm below the elbow with the opposite hand, pushing hard towards the elbows without moving either hand up the arm (see Fig. 8.3).
● To *exercise the waist*, stand with legs apart (i.e. 9 ins/23 cm) and the arms raised above the head. Ensure that the posture is maintained and make alternate bends from the waist to the left and to the right (see Fig. 8.4).
● To *strengthen abdominal muscles*, lie in a supine position (i.e. on the back), raise one leg at an angle off the floor and hold to the count of five. Then continue to raise the leg as high as possible and again count to five before lowering the leg very slowly to the floor. This should be repeated with the other leg (see Fig. 8.5(a) and (b)).
● To *firm the thighs*, lie on one side with the head supported by an arm and the other hand on the floor in front of the waist. Lift the outside leg as high as possible, keeping the toes pointed and hold to the count of five, then lower the leg very slowly. Turn to the other side and repeat the exercise (see Fig. 8.6).

● *Cycling* is very good for the *legs*. Lie in a supine position with hands at the sides and lift the legs from the hips and 'cycle', ensuring that the back is kept flat on the floor. The toes should brush the floor as they come down (see Fig. 8.7).

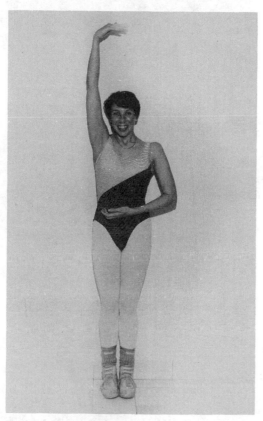

Fig. 8.1 Super-stretch

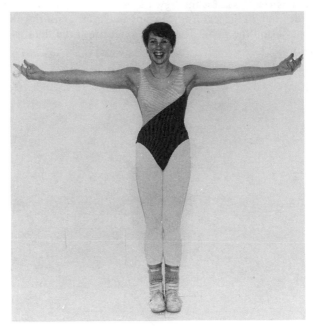

Fig. 8.2 Hand circling

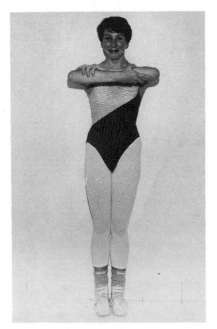

Fig. 8.3 Firming the bust

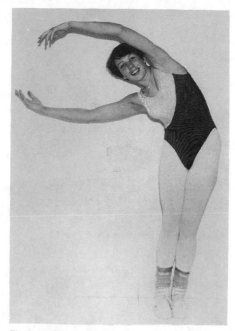

Fig. 8.4 Bends to the side to exercise the waist

(a)

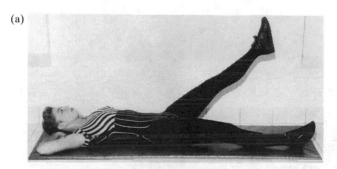

(b)

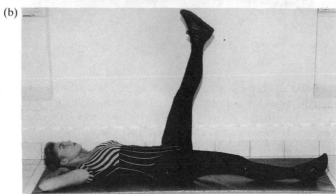

Fig. 8.5 (a) Raising leg to strengthen abdominal muscles
(b) Raising leg as high as possible to strengthen abdominal muscles

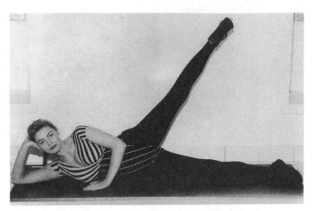

Fig. 8.6 Raising leg to the side to firm thigh muscles

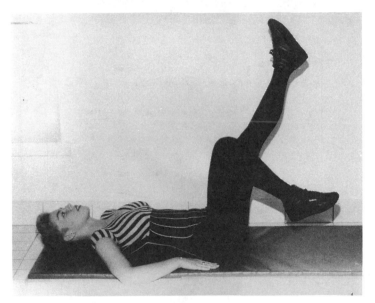

Fig. 8.7 'Cycling' movement

The repetition of each exercise is at the discretion of the beauty therapist. They are not strenuous and can be carried out by most clients. It is important to interrupt the programme occasionally to allow for postural correction, to repeat breathing exercises and check the pulse rate.

After the exercise period, do not stop suddenly but use 'warm-down' exercises and try to finish with a relaxation technique.

Movements to avoid

There are movements that can cause injury to the body and these should be avoided. For example:

- when circling the head, ensure that the client does not *hold* the head backwards as this contracts the back muscles of the neck which are probably very tight and increases the probability of damaging the intervertebral discs in the cervical area;
- do not hyper-extend any joint, e.g. locking the knees or elbows. The knees are especially vulnerable as locking puts a great deal of stress on the ligaments supporting the knee joint (this also applies to the elbows);
- at the same time, over-bending of the knees, that is where the knee-bend is too deep, shifts the body-weight from the thigh muscles to the knee ligaments which causes considerable strain on the latter;
- when 'bicycling' the legs, always ensure that the back is flat on the floor; never raise the body on to the neck for this exercise, as excess pressure will be put on to the intervertebral discs;
- when lying with the back on the floor, never lift both legs up straight and then lower them to the floor. This exercise was supposed to strengthen the abdominal muscles, but in effect the weight of the legs usually forces the back into an arched position, causing considerable strain on the back;
- be careful when giving exercises for the waist to ensure that the spine is not subjected to repeated bending forward and backward, again to avoid any pressure on the lower back.

There are other 'no-go' exercises and the therapist must think through the planned programme to ensure that it is completely safe.

If taking a class, the therapist should ensure that interest is stimulated and maintained by having a cheerful voice giving good exercise commands and, where possible, using music to suit the programme. It is usual to find the music, adapt it to the exercise routine and then put it on 'tape' for future use. It is amazing how quickly a library of tapes can be built up for different types of exercises, i.e. special exercises for specific problems; balance and exercise sequences; relaxation techniques.

Home exercises should be shown and practised with the client and followed up at the next session.

Types of exercise

There are many types of exercises and most of them can be incorporated in one session which will give variety and avoid boredom. One chapter could not possibly cover this subject and beauty therapists are advised to read some of the numerous books published which give a wide range of exercises together with variations.

Isotonic exercise

Isotonic exercises involve active movements where limbs are moved and the muscles concerned change in shape and length; the involuntary muscles of the heart and circulatory system are strengthened. Most general exercise will be of the isotonic, free flowing type, improving suppleness, body shape, respiration and circulation.

Aerobic exercise

Aerobic exercise is a variation on the isotonic technique. It is the name given to the practice of maintaining an isotonic exercise at a strenuous level for a minimum length of time. It is the type of exercise which improves the cardiovascular fitness and increases stamina. It covers any exercises that make the heart pump faster than normal and make breathing deeper and more rapid so that the lungs are used to maximum capacity. All aerobics involve large muscle groups, primarily those of the hips and legs and include jogging, swimming, cycling, running, walking and many social sports, i.e. tennis, golf, etc. Therefore, aerobic exercises do not necessarily tone up muscles all over the body, nor do they help suppleness. Very popular now are 'aerobic classes' which involve a mixture of dance and exercise and, if taught properly, can be sustained for over five minutes.

It is essential for the client to work out a training level, i.e. the rate at which the heart should be beating during exercise in order to have a beneficial effect. The heart should be beating from approximately 60–80 per cent of its safe maximum. The therapist should always be observant, looking for telltale signs of over-exertion, e.g. breathlessness, or an unusually red or pale complexion, in which case the client has probably misread the pulse check and has exceeded his/her aerobic capacity.

Isometric exercise

This is a group of exercises that can be carried out by most groups of people, fit and unfit, ill and well, old and young, arthritic and disabled. Isometric contraction refers to the tensing or tightening of a muscle without changing its length and has a benefit in increasing the tone of voluntary muscles but has no effect on involuntary muscles. Very little fatigue results so *most* of the exercises are suitable for clients with heart or lung complaints or with any other contra-indications which prevent a normal active exercise routine. However, care must be taken to select the correct exercises. To have the best effect, the contraction of each muscle must be carried out with complete mental concentration and held for a full six seconds, while breathing naturally, before being released.

A few resistive exercises are given where the maximum tension should be held for 3 to 6 seconds. These can be shown to the client and also used as simple home exercises.

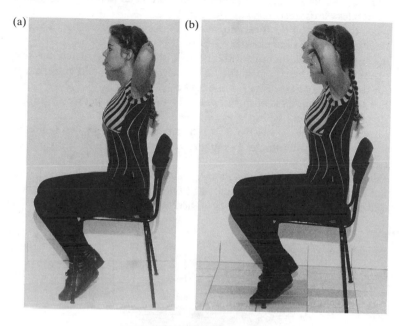

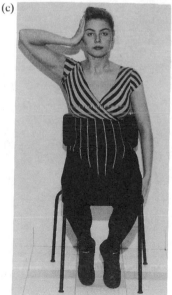

Fig. 8.8 (a) Exercises for the neck muscles – trying to force head backwards
(b) Exercises for the neck muscles – trying to push head forward
(c) Exercises for the neck muscles – trying to push the head sideways

Exercises sitting on a chair

- For *neck muscles*, place the hands behind the head and try to force the head backwards, resisting with the arms;
- place the hands on the forehead and try to push the head forward (again resisting with the arms); and
- place one hand on the side of the head, with the other grasping the seat of the chair, and try to push the head sideways; this should be repeated for the other side (see Fig. 8.8 a, b and c).
- For the *chest muscles*, push the palms of the hands together to form a strong contraction (see Fig. 8.9).
- Sit with a cushion on the lap. Grip the sides of the chair then bend the knees and raise the thighs to squeeze the cushion against the stomach (see Fig. 8.10).
- For *shoulder muscles*, sit on an armless chair with the palms of the hands flat on the seat and arms straight. Lift buttocks and thighs off the chair and feet off the floor. This will be difficult for the unfit (see Fig. 8.11).

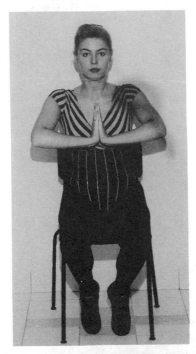

Fig. 8.9 Exercises for the chest muscles – pushing the palms of the hands together

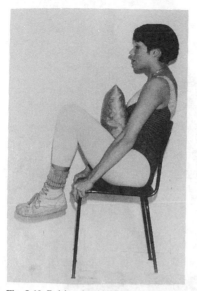

Fig. 8.10 Raising the thighs to squeeze the
cushion against the stomach

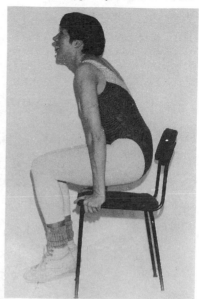

Fig. 8.11 Lifting the buttocks and thighs off the cha

Exercises lying on the floor, supine position

● For *neck muscles*, push the back of the head down (see Fig. 8.12).
● For *chest muscles*, lift the bust, pressing the hands down on the floor as
hard as possible.
● For the *waist and abdominal muscles*, bend the knees with the soles of
the feet firmly on the floor, place hands behind the head and bring the
shoulders off the floor. Progression would be to raise the body to a sitting
position (see Fig. 8.13),
● For the *thigh muscles*, cross the ankles and try to pull the feet apart (see
Fig. 8.14) or again cross the ankles and lift the bottom leg up and press
the top leg down.
● For the *calf muscles*, squeeze a cushion between the ankles, at the same
time turning the toes inwards. Repeat turning the toes outward (see Fig.
8.15).

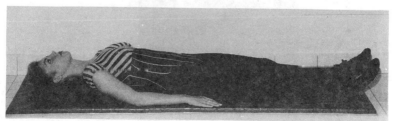

Fig. 8.12 For the neck muscles, push the back of the head down on to the floor

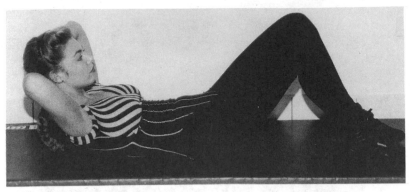

Fig. 8.13 For waist and abdominal muscles, bringing the shoulders off the floor

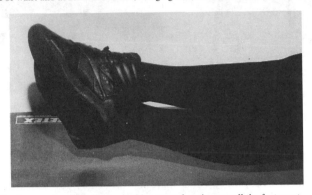

Fig. 8.14 For the muscles of the thighs – ankles crossed, trying to pull the feet apart

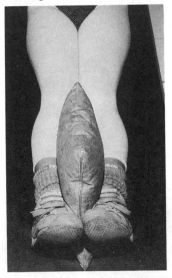

Fig. 8.15 Squeezing a cushion between ankles and turning the toes inwards

Exercises in the standing position

● To *increase or firm the bust*, place the hands on each side of a door at eye level. Press as hard as possible and repeat with hands at chest level and then at waist level (see Fig. 8.16).

● To *firm the waist and hips*, stand sideways 12–18 in (30–45 cm) away from a wall and place the outside hand over the head and push against the wall with the palm of the hand. Reverse the body and use the other hand (see Fig. 8.17).

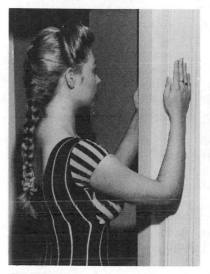

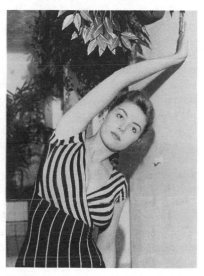

Fig. 8.16 To firm the bust – starting with the hands each side of the door frame (at eye level)

Fig. 8.17 To firm waist – pushing against the wall with the palm of the hand

Callisthenic exercise

Callisthenic exercises are really an extension of isometric exercise, incorporating a few isotonic movements to build up strength and suppleness to improve the shape of the body. They do not lead to all-round fitness as they do not improve the condition of the heart or lungs.

Yoga

The aim of yoga, which has been practised for centuries in the East, is to increase the body's suppleness and mobility and ultimately to achieve deep mental relaxation. It is a specialised form of exercise which requires considerable tuition.

Exercise machines

The use of exercise machines creates variety but clients should always be supervised to ensure that they are used correctly. In purchasing any piece of equipment, demonstration and advice must be obtained from the supplier. The following are a few examples.

Stationary exercise bicycles   have long been part of the exercise industry and they perform the same movements as those of the 'real' activity. However, for all their end results, they can be extremely boring. Manufacturers are now concentrating on variations and improvements, i.e. ergometers, whereby the resistance of the pedals can be adjusted, a gauge to show the distance covered and some machines register the speed at which the pedals are pushed round and calculate the energy expended in either Kjoules /KM or calories/mile. More progressive designs and technological innovation offer a computer video screen which precisely simulates features of a countryside ride such as gradients, speed, frictions and wind resistance.

The jogging machine   resembles a short conveyor belt, where the client runs 'on the spot' on the moving surface. The speed is adjusted to the running capability of the client so that he/she does not run off the front or fall off the back. The machine measures the distance covered, speed and time taken.

The rowing machine   also simulates the 'real' activity. There is a bar against which the feet are braced and two levers, one for each hand, resembling the oars of a rowing boat. As with bicycle pedals, the resistance of these 'oars' can be adjusted.

Weights   vary from hand-held weights to a dumb-bell or a solid metal disc balanced on a cross bar, with adjustable weights. These are mainly used for weight training which involves lifting a weight slowly and smoothly several times. There are also available weighted bands which can be worn around the ankles or wrists and these make the muscles of the legs or arms, shoulders and chest work much harder. However, these should not be worn during warm-up exercises.

Skipping rope   the simplest way to fitness. It is unlikely that your area will be large enough for this activity but clients can be advised to do this at home – in the garden or on a terrace.

Toning tables   are being extensively used to improve postural deficiencies. Toning restores the physiological conditions through several mechanisms, e.g. tensed muscles are relaxed by vibration; using passive movements, joints regain their original flexibility; active resistance against the tables' movement will increase muscle strength. Therefore, regular use will not only help to restore a normal posture but maintain it. Passive use of the toning tables is good for the elderly disabled and vastly overweight.

Water exercises

Swimming has been considered as the best all-round sport of keeping fit but water exercises can have the same benefits as swimming whether the client knows how to swim or not. The key to toning muscles and shaping the body is working against resistance. Water, due to its buoyancy properties, offers enormous resistance – twelve times as much as air – but feels almost effortless because of the lack of gravitational pull. Very few clients will have their own pool and will need to rely on public swimming pools or pools located in leisure clubs. Pools come in various shapes and sizes, especially when it comes to the shallowest and deepest depths and the holding-on facilities. The latter may be in the form of a ladder, steps or a holding rail which are ideal for certain exercises and for the non-swimmers. Try and find an area for the client/s where the water comes to the waist or chest area when the feet are on the bottom of the pool.

The sequence of the exercises will depend on the temperature of the pool. Ideally stretching exercises come first, followed by warm-up exercises and then flexing exercises. However, if the water is cool, start with warm-up exercises with the client standing with the water at waist level and use any exercise that includes walking or running through the water or bouncing up and down (see Fig. 8.18).

Stretching exercises involve muscles and joints, and the following exercises are for the arms, waist and thighs.

Arms   in shoulder-depth water (either standing or having knees bent) with the arms at the sides of the body and back straight, use the palms as oars and

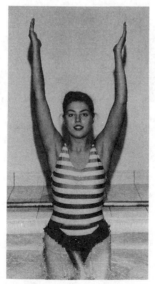

Fig. 8.18 Warm-up exercises – bouncing up and down in the water

pull the arms upwards to the surface of the water and down again to the sides. This can be followed by bending the arm across in front of the chest with the palm facing the body. Straighten the elbow and push the arm back against the water. This exercise also benefits the muscles of the shoulders and chest (see Fig. 8.19).

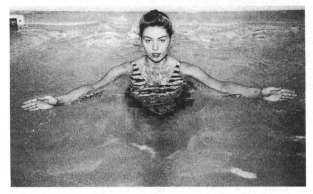

Fig. 8.19 Stretching exercises for the arms – pushing the arms back against the water

Waist   preferably with water at level of the midriff, stand with legs apart for balance and place hands on the hips. Turn from the waist to the right and to the left, keeping the elbows back at all times (see Fig. 8.20).

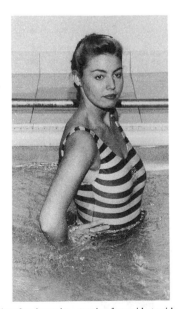

Fig. 8.20 Stretching exercises for the waist – turning from side to side in the water

Thighs in at least waist-depth of water, extend arms sideways and raise one knee out to the side and as high as possible. Try to touch the arm with the knee, keeping the back straight and facing the front. Repeat with the other knee. This may be difficult at first, but the same exercise can be done with one hand holding the side of the pool (see Fig. 8.21).

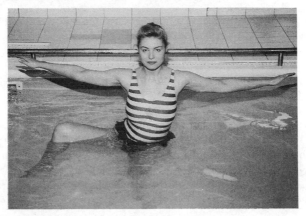

Fig. 8.21 Stretching exercises for the thighs – extending arms and raising one knee out to the side, as high as possible

Flexing exercises tone up the body generally and are more fitness-orientated incorporating endurance, strength and resilience.

See also Chapter 9 (Fig. 9.4) showing water exercises with the whirlpool in the background.

Therapists taking a class can, in time, progress the clients to a more difficult programme by repetition and an increase in depth of water.

Specific exercises

The obese client

The exercise plan for the obese client has to be worked out very carefully with advice given on dietary control. Many clients will have very large thighs and are unable to cross their legs or have difficulty in lowering themselves to the floor and getting up again. Initially, exercises performed on a chair or standing will have more benefit.

Neck area all the isometric exercises detailed in Fig. 8.8 sitting on a chair (preferably armless) will help to strengthen and mobilise the area.

Shoulders area use a standing position and give various arm movements, i.e. elbow circling, where the arms are bent at the elbows and rotated inwards and outwards and forward and backwards; swinging the arms backwards and forwards together and then alternately; swinging an arm across the chest and out to the side at shoulder level.

Bust   pressing the hands together as seen in Fig. 8.3 strengthens the pectoral muscles.

Waist   simple, alternate bends to the sides of the body followed by trunk turning, where the client places her hands behind the head and turns to the right and to the left without moving the hips.

Stomach   posture, deep breathing and isometric exercises are advised until the client becomes fitter.

Hips   initially the best exercise is walking or, in the salon, bench stepping. Ensure your bench is wide and firm and show the client how to step up and down with alternate feet. Although this is an exercise for general strengthening of the legs it does move the hip joint, improving mobility. When the client is able to lie or sit comfortably on the floor there are many more exercises that can be given.

Thighs and legs   again advise walking but in the salon exercises can be given to improve mobility, i.e. high stepping, whereby alternate knees are lifted towards the chest, slowly at first but gradually increasing the speed; or jogging on the spot. However, it should be remembered that the knee joints are carrying a great deal of weight so the exercises should not be carried out for long periods at a time.

Most water exercises can be accomplished by obese clients and all exercises can be progressed as the client's mobility improves.

During and after pregnancy

Ante-natal and post-natal clinics give considerable advice on exercises and the therapist can ensure that the client maintains her programme throughout. Liaison with these clinics is obviously beneficial. Posture and breathing need special attention during pregnancy. Advise the client when sitting to have adequate back support and put the feet up when possible. Exercises to circle the ankles to help prevent oedema and foot arching to strengthen the arch of the foot should be given. When standing advise the client to keep her weight evenly distributed, neither leaning forward on the balls of the feet or swaying backwards on the heels, as this is a great temptation as pregnancy advances and the balance changes. Good, deep, slow breathing is also important.

During pregnancy the client is likely to put on approximately 18–20 lb (8.1–9 kg) in weight and this is made up by:

weight of the average baby	7 lb (3.2kg)
weight of the placenta	1½ lb (675g)

weight of the amniotic fluid	2 lb (900g)
weight of the uterus	2 lb (900g)
increased blood volume	4 lb (1.8kg)
increased volume of the breasts	1½ lb (675g)
Totalling	18 lb (8.1kg)

There could also be extra fluid retention but the client should be advised to keep her weight gain within reason and not exceed 28 lb (12.6kg).

Breasts enlarge during pregnancy, and exercises to strengthen the pectoral muscles should be advised.

Exercises for the abdominal and pelvic floor muscles will be given by the clinic as strong muscles make for an easier delivery.

Following the birth, medical post-natal exercises are given. Once the post-natal examination has taken place, which is usually six weeks after the birth, the client can begin exercises in the salon. She is normally anxious to regain her figure, but with new responsibilities it is often difficult for her to find the time for regular exercise and visits to the salon. Encouragement should be given with exercises to strengthen the abdominal muscles and improve the general slackness of the body. Commence the programme slowly with gentle isometric exercises for the abdomen and isotonic exercises for the waist, i.e. side-bending and trunk rotation with the arms outstretched and for the thighs, bicycling, walking etc. Explain that the two can be combined when taking the baby out in the pram, i.e. retraction of the abdominal muscles while walking.

Stress

Stress and its partner, tension, manifest themselves in a number of different ways: irritability, hunching of the shoulders, headaches, backaches etc., for which there is no physiological reason. Drugs only bring temporary relief; the clients really have to eradicate the source of the tension, which is primarily the result of unresolved inner conflict. The therapist can help by teaching them to relax both mind and muscle.

Probably the best method of relaxation is based on 'tense a muscle and let it go' technique. For this routine an area in the salon that is very quiet should be found. The client should lie in a supine position initially and covered with a blanket to retain warmth. Start with rhythmical deep breathing, in through the nose and out through the mouth, which should be partially opened with the jaw relaxed. The therapist should talk quietly and explain that the whole body is going to be tensed and relaxed, by letting each area literally 'flop', beginning with the feet:

● point the toes to the floor, relax; bring the toes to point up to the ceiling, relax;
● push the heels down to tighten the calf muscles, relax; and so continue up the legs, using groups of muscles to tense and relax.

This is followed by:

- the clenching and relaxing of the buttocks;
- retraction and relaxation of the abdomen;
- clenching the fists, and tensing the muscle groups of the arms and relaxing these;
- pressing the shoulder blades into the floor/couch and relax;
- pursing the mouth, screwing up the face and letting go completes the routine.

The number of times each muscle is tensed is irrelevant, but it is important to give a quiet, slow, rhythmical instruction.

At the end of the relaxation routine, the client may have fallen asleep or wish to change to a more comfortable position. Let the client rest, and if asleep, allowed to wake-up naturally. Busy salons rarely have the time or space available but if the client can be taught just once, it will prove invaluable for them to practise at home.

Chapter 9

Pre-heating the tissues

Some form of heat treatment is given in most salons where body services are given. Heat relaxes body tissue and tense muscles and by pre-heating the tissues, prior to massage or electrical therapy, it improves the effectiveness of these treatments. There are various forms of heat therapy available but whichever type is chosen it must be remembered that it is dangerous to increase the body temperature more than two or three degrees.

Sauna

A sauna, which is based on the Finnish principle of a log cabin, can be made to any size, according to the needs of the salon. However, it is important that the area is large enough, has adequate ventilation and is preferably sited on the ground floor to minimise any fire risk. As a very rough guide to space, a minimum of 64 sq.ft (6 sq.m) would be required for the smallest two-seater sauna, a shower unit, a changing cubicle and rest area.

There are two types of sauna available, i.e. a *panel sauna*, which is made of two panels of wood, usually pine, with a layer of insulating material between the panels, or the more traditional *log sauna*, which uses solid wood, usually thick lengths of pine, slightly curved on each side to resemble logs. Both are free-standing units and should be erected on an even floor of quarry tiles or non-slip ceramic tiles, or even a sheet of vinyl, although the latter often warps with the heat.

Sauna fittings include vents, i.e. air outlet and inlet vents, a thermostat, benches, usually at two levels, a guard rail for the stove, duckboards for the floor, sauna pail and a long handled ladle. The light inside the cabin must be insulated and protected to prevent breakage or an accidental burn. There should be an observation window in the door and a buzzer or a bell in the sauna. A clock or timer can be very useful (see Fig. 9.1).

The air within the sauna is changed about six times an hour, and all the moisture within is removed, so that the air is prevented from becoming stale and the sauna unhygienic.

No special plumbing is required for the sauna itself, but it should be sited where there is a supply of hot and cold water and a drainage system for a

Window

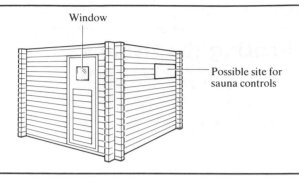

Possible site for
sauna controls

Fig. 9.1 Sauna

shower. Hosing down the sauna, scrubbing and rinsing the wooden benches (which must be carried out at regular intervals) or cleaning the area is made much easier if there is a channel to a drain located near the sauna. Detergents should not be used as these can be absorbed by the wood, creating a smell, but more importantly the wood in time would rot.

The electricity required is dependent upon the size of the sauna. The heat in the sauna is produced by an electric heater in a stove with special stones which are placed on a tray on top of the stove. Small 3 kilowatt stoves (i.e. a sauna for 2–3 persons) can operate off a normal 13 amp ring main, but larger stoves (i.e. 4 to 9 kilowatts) require more power and a special cable which must be connected to a control box by a qualified electrician. For safety reasons, this connection should be well away from the area. If possible, to prevent interference by clients to alter the temperature in the sauna, this control should be outside the cabin.

To heat up the sauna cabin completely will take between 30 and 60 minutes, dependent on the size. When the set temperature has been reached, the thermostat, inside the cabin, will operate and cut off the power temporarily until required again. The special stones emit the heat which rises on convection currents and although the heat produced is indirect it becomes constant. When the walls of the sauna have absorbed all the heat possible, it is radiated back into the cabin.

The temperature in the sauna should induce free sweating; it is pointless to subject the body to any temperature higher than this. Women usually prefer a sauna at 60–70°C (140–158°F) whereas men prefer a temperature of 80–90°C (176–194°F). The sauna is a dry heat but slight humidity can be produced by ladling water (from the sauna pail) on to the stones.

The effects of a sauna

● Stimulates blood circulation, increases pulse rate and raises body temperature.

Effect on blood pressure is variable, but commonly falls due to the heat and relaxation.

● Heat helps to activate over two million sweat glands in the skin. Therefore mineral salts and other substances, including toxins, normally excreted by the kidneys, are discharged through the dilated pores of the skin. The result of this elimination means that the skin is thoroughly cleansed – pores unblocked and blackheads loosened – and is in a much healthier condition.

Minor aches and pains will be relieved, stiff joints are loosened and tissues are softened.

Temporary water weight loss may ensue due to dehydration during the time spent in the sauna but this is replaced as soon as the client drinks (water or tea).

Contra-indications

Cardio-vascular conditions i.e. angina pectoris or a history of thrombosis, varicose veins;
● abnormally high or low blood pressure;
any congestive condition of the lungs (i.e. asthma);
● skin diseases (with the exception of acne vulgaris) oedema and inflammation;
● epilepsy;
● diabetes;
during the first two days of menstruation if the client is not well or suffers from cramps;
● during pregnancy;
within two or three hours of a heavy meal;
● under the influence of drink;
● severe exhaustion;
● migraine;
● liver, kidney and pancreatic disorders, without doctor's permission;
elderly clients, without doctor's permission;
skin infections, i.e. tinea pedis, verrucae or plantar warts, unless the client wears adequate protection in the sauna and throughout the treatment area.

Contra-indications are important as people have died in saunas, so it is wise to display a notice detailing these, either at the reception desk or on the outside of the sauna. However, if a client takes a sauna, or in fact any other treatment, contrary to the advice of the therapist, he/she must sign an indemnity against any ill effects to release the therapist from responsibility. The following is a suggestion for the type of indemnity form which could be used:

[Name of the salon]

I, the undersigned, freely accept that I am not complying with the advice and recommendations, listed below, which will be given to me by the therapeutic staff of this salon. I further accept that [name of salon] and their staff shall in no way whatsoever be held responsible for any ill-effects, damage (to the person or property) or injury that may be suffered by me, or be caused by me, as a result of not complying with the said advice and recommendations.

Signed: [client] ....

Name: (in block letters) [client] ....

Address: ....

    ....

Date: ....

Recommendations: ....

    ....

    ....

This form was presented to: ....

on . . . . . . date . . . . by . . . . [therapist] . . . .

Signed by . . . . [therapist]

Method of use

- Complete a record card and check for any contra-indication. If the therapist has any doubts about the health of the client, pulse and blood pressure should be taken.
- Client undresses and showers with warm water and liquid soap. (Do not use a bar of soap which has to be shared among the clients as this is unhygienic.) As well as the body, the head will perspire so make-up should be removed and advise brushing the hair if lacquer is used as this will become sticky with the heat in the sauna. Request the client to remove any jewellery as it can heat up rapidly, causing a 'hot-spot' and may cause a burn. Also make sure that the *client* puts the jewellery away safely. In an ideal situation a salon would have sufficient space for lockers with keys for clients, but usually jewellery/watches are put into handbags or trousers.
- Give the client towels, one to wrap around the body and another to place on the bench.
- Advise the client to sit on the lower bench initially until he/she becomes used to the heat and to breathe with the mouth open.
- After about ten minutes the client should take a *tepid* shower, no soap, and this cycle can be repeated as often as the client wishes or time permits. The client may also progress to a higher bench to gain more heat and/or put water on the stones to give humidity.
- When the sauna treatment is complete the client should wash in the shower and, if no further treatment follows, relax for about 15 minutes before dressing and leaving the salon.

The sauna is expensive to run but can be shared with other clients. A few salons provide birch twigs which are used to increase circulation but these are difficult to keep clean.

Hygiene should be observed at all times, not only with the sauna but within the entire area. Safety is an important factor. Ensure that the area does not become slippery. Display notices to advise clients to dry their feet after a shower and, if needed, use duckboards from the shower to the sauna. Clients should not be left unattended – a person may faint or fall, or simply fall asleep in the sauna. If a client looks unwell, enter the sauna, leave the door wide open for air and, if necessary, help the client out of the sauna to the relaxation area and give sips of cold water. To prevent the risk of fire, clients should not be allowed to take magazines, books or newspapers into the sauna. Ensure that there are adequate waste-bins, and laundry baskets for used towels.

Small niceties are always appreciated and cost very little, i.e. shower caps, box of tissues, a large jug of water with ice and slices of lemon or orange, plastic glasses (not glass, in case of breakage), a moisturiser and talcum powder. Coin-operated hair-dryers are always useful, but it depends on the area as these can be quite noisy.

Steam cabinet

The steam cabinet is a very popular form of pre-heating the body as it takes up less room than the sauna, can be plugged into a 13 amp ring main and is much cheaper to run. However, it can only take one client at a time.

The cabinet itself is usually made of fibreglass, the old metal steam cabinets having more or less disappeared now (see Fig. 9.2). Most cabinets have one door (with a curved aperture for the neck) which either opens to the side or drops forward, supported by small chains. The seat inside can usually be adjusted so that the client can sit comfortably and allow the head to be free from the cabinet.

Steam is produced by a small horse-shoe shaped electrical element heating the water in a container just below the seat. Above the container is a thermostat probe which is connected to a dial on the outside of the cabinet. The container itself has a cover which should be fitted properly to provide protection for the client's legs and allow the steam to circulate freely in the cabinet. To fill the container with water, remove the cover, and use a watering can, preferably with a long spout.

Care should be taken not to knock the probe of the thermostat out of alignment before replacing the cover in position. Also outside the cabinet there is a timer which is usually used in conjunction with the thermostat to provide the client with the heat and time required for the treatment. There are cabinets which have free-standing seats and these must be covered with a towel to protect the client from direct steam.

Dependent on the size of the container, the water will probably take 15–20 minutes (i.e. from cold) to reach the required temperature. Steam cabinet temperatures are invariably lower because steam will scald, being a wet heat whereas the sauna is a dry heat. The treatment can last for 20 minutes on a low heat i.e. 33°C (92°F) or a maximum of 5–10 minutes on a high heat, i.e. 48°C (118°F).

The effects of a steam cabinet

● There is no noticeable rise in body temperature or pulse rate.
  Heats the body resulting in an increase in circulation.
  Promotes sebaceous and sudoriferous gland activity.
● Relaxes and softens the body tissues, relieves minor aches and pains and loosens stiff joints.

Contra-indications

Heart conditions, abnormally high or low blood pressure;
thrombosis;
diabetes;
epilepsy;
skin diseases (as with sauna);
renal disorders (as with sauna);
skin infections (as with sauna);

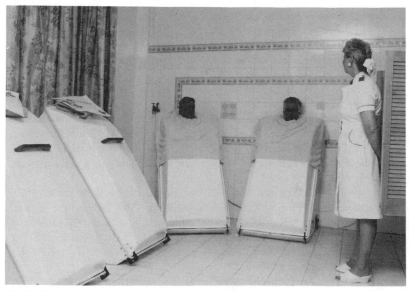

Fig. 9.2 Steam cabinets

- under the influence of drink or less than two hours after a heavy meal;
- severe exhaustion.

These contra-indications are very similar to those given for the sauna. However, there are instances whereby a steam cabinet on a low heat may be given. For instance, a client who suffers from asthma can often take a steam bath; because the head remains outside the cabinet, he/she is able to breathe in atmospheric air; clients with slight varicose veining can also take a steam bath without any ill effect; psoriasis can actually be helped by the wet heat; migraine sufferers can often tolerate a steam bath, whereas the sauna may trigger off an attack. It is a matter which requires a great deal of common sense from the therapist, watching client reaction very carefully and terminating the treatment if the client appears at all unwell.

Method of use

Before the client arrives, ensure that the container is full of water (it usually takes about 3–4 litres (or ¾–1 gallon) and replace the cover. Place a paper bath mat on the floor of the cabinet, drape a towel over the seat taking it up over the back of the cabinet (or use paper towels on the seat), close the door and place another towel over the aperture. Push the plug of the steam cabinet into the ring main and switch on. Rotate the dials of the thermostat and the timer to the required heat and time. This applies to most steam cabinets but there are other types where the manufacturer's instructions should be followed.

- When the client arrives, complete a record card and check for any contra-indications.
- As with a sauna treatment, all jewellery etc. should be removed and put away safely.
- Request the client to undress and while he/she is showering (with warm water and liquid soap), check the temperature of the steam cabinet and that the seat is securely supported and at the correct height.
- Ensure that the client's feet are dry when leaving the shower and use a towel to wrap around the body to go to the cabinet. This towel can be used as a screen as the client enters the cabinet (especially if there are other people in the area) before placing in the laundry basket.
- Remove the towel from the aperture, assist the client into the cabinet, close the door and wrap this towel around the client's neck to prevent any steam escaping. Check the timer, the thermostat will maintain the temperature selected by switching on and off automatically. The therapist must always supervise the client taking a steam bath.
- Explain to the client how easy it is to push the door open. This will alleviate any anxiety the client may have of being restricted and it also allows heat to escape quickly should the temperature in the cabinet become uncomfortable.

- If the excess moisture appears on the client's brow or tip of the nose this should be removed with a tissue by the therapist.
- When the treatment time has lapsed (usually between 15 and 20 minutes) remove the towel from the neck and use this to wrap around the body for the client to go to the shower.
- Ensure the shower water is warm, the client should wash well with liquid soap to remove the sweat. Body scrubs or sea salt rubs are useful to remove dead surface skin. Hand the client a towel to rub dry.
- If no further treatment follows, the client should relax for about 15 minutes to allow skin temperature to return to normal before dressing and leaving the salon.

Remove the towel from inside the cabinet and dispose of the paper bath mat/s and wipe the area with an antiseptic lotion. Always check the level of water in the container after each client and essences may be added to the water to produce a pleasant smell. To prevent stagnant water odour the container should be emptied and rinsed with clean water at the end of the day and the floor of the cabinet should be dried with a cloth to avoid sediment formation. The steam cabinet is best left open overnight. Again, similar to the sauna, clients will appreciate small amenities.

Steam rooms

The social centres of years ago where people met and relaxed were the Turkish rooms which had a traditional mix of steam rooms, hot rooms, and plunge pools. There are a few left in the UK which have been carefully modernised but retaining their original concept.

Modern steam rooms are usually available as a ready-for-assembly package where the walls, ceiling and seats are made in glass-fibre reinforced plastic. The domed ceiling and curved back rests ensure that the condensation runs down the walls to the floor. They can be installed on floors of brick or non-slip tiles but must have a drain outlet within the steam room and larger units are usually found in hydros/spas or leisure centres where there is plenty of room.

Steam is provided from a generator that can be mounted outside the steam room (see Fig. 9.3) or located in a cupboard anywhere within 13 yards (12 m) of the steam room. It requires connection to the mains electrical supply, hot and cold running water and, of course, the drain outlet. The master control panel, which includes an on/off switch, timer and thermostatic control, is mounted on a wall where the therapist can best manage them. An aromatic injector can also be placed beside this panel. These larger steam rooms will also require an air inlet and outlet vents fitted. Some manufacturers can also supply an automatic disinfectant system via spreaders to disinfect seats and walls when the steam room is unoccupied.

The ambient temperature inside the room should not exceed 49°C (120°F)

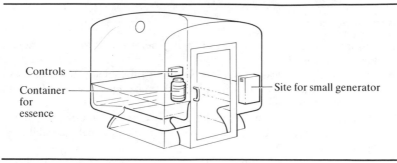

Controls

Container
for
essence

Site for small generator

Fig. 9.3 Steam Room

and the therapist should provide an accurate thermometer (so that clients may check the temperature before entering) and a clock or timer inside so that clients may time their stay.

However, there are smaller units available for 1–2 people taking up less than 212 cu. ft (6 cu. m) in size which could be useful for salons. The same equipment is needed but the generator would be smaller and there would not be a requirement for ventilation. Also available are shower cabinets with a steam facility, i.e. a shower with sprinkler head, a moulded plastic seat and a small generator outside the cubicle.

The effects of the steam room

The effects are similar to those of the steam cabinet with the combination of heat and humidity increasing circulation and for the therapeutic effect on muscular aches and pains.

Contra-indications

Contra-indications are the same as those for the sauna/steam cabinets and again it is wise to display notices advising the clients of these. Where these steam rooms are part of a leisure centre, many clients may have taken part in a hard aerobic workout just prior to entering the steam room; this will mean that the clients are already 'well-heated', even if a cool-down period has allowed the heart rate to return to a safe level. The therapist should ensure that ample time is allowed for the overall temperature of the body to drop to a normal level. It should be remembered that, unlike the sauna where heat is more easily dissipated, in the damp conditions of the steam room sweat does not easily evaporate. In consequence, skin and body temperature rise and the steam room feels hotter than a sauna because the steam serves to prevent sweat evaporating easily and also because the humid air stores more heat than the dry air in a sauna.

Method of use

- Ensure there is plenty of water in the generator and that the ambient temperature is reached.
- Take the same precautions as for sauna/steam cabinets and also make sure that clients are not wearing jewellery, make-up or using body oils as these inhibit sweating.
- Request the client to shower with liquid soap before entering the room.
- Give the client a towel (on which to sit) to avoid any slight possibility of bacterial contamination.
- Make frequent checks through the door/window to ensure that clients are comfortable. Advise clients that if they experience any discomfort at all, i.e. nausea or headache, dizziness, hot or cold chills, they should leave the steam room immediately.
- Ensure that towels are handy when they leave the room to shower.

Always suggest warm or tepid showers as very cold showers or ice-cold water in a plunge pool will increase the peripheral resistance and greatly elevate blood pressure.

Hygiene and safety should be observed at all times and clients advised to rest (if no further treatment follows) for 15–20 minutes before dressing.

Whirlpools

These are mentioned here briefly as they are usually found in leisure centres or hydros/spas. The baths come in all shapes and sizes and are made from strong laminate reinforced with glass fibres. The inside of the bath is curved to form seats, usually at varying heights. As the whirlpool is a mixture of air and water, jets are placed below the water level (the number of which is dependent on the size of the bath). The pump and various mechanical equipment connected to the bath is either stored beneath the bath or in a separate cupboard nearby.

The water inside the whirlpool is kept at approximately 37.8°C (100°F) and to prevent bacterial growth the water needs to be continually chemically treated to maintain a high standard of hygiene. In most cases this can be carried out automatically. One of the reasons why owners of a small salon should think very carefully about the installation of a whirlpool is the considerable amount of condensation arising and the effect it has on the surroundings even when humidifiers and extractor fans are installed. Fig. 9.4 shows a whirlpool at the rear of a pool area.

The controls on the ledge of the bath comprise a timer, which is usually set for 10–15 minutes, and a dial for regulating the force of air into the water through the jets.

In a commercial situation the chemical dosage is fairly high and it is wise to display notices giving advice on the use of the whirlpool, e.g.

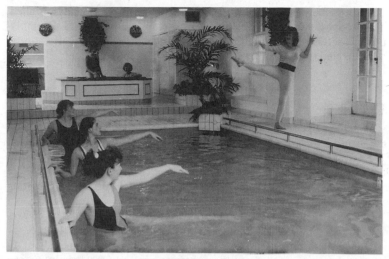

Fig. 9.4 Whirlpool at the end of the pool area

- contra-indications, which are the same as for the steam and sauna baths and severe exhaustion;
- clients should be advised to shower before and after the use of the bath;
- the use of the whirlpool should be limited initially to 10 minutes, as it can be quite exhausting;
- the dial for the jets should be at a setting which would be comfortable for most clients;
- clients with bleached hair should wear a shower cap as in some instances the hair can turn 'green'!

Hygiene and safety must be considered at all times. At the end of the day the whirlpool should be emptied, cleaned and refilled with water, together with the appropriate chemicals, and covered to retain heat and save energy.

Spa baths

A rather misused word, as spa usually means a mineral spring or a resort where such springs exist but it is assumed that it means a bath which is aerated, which could also apply to the whirlpool! Hydrotherapy baths can be considered as spa baths providing the hoses used for massage are put to one side and the jets on the side of the bath are used to aerate the water. Additives, such as foaming agents, seaweed and peat, heighten the effects of relaxation. If the salon has an area large enough for a standard bath, there are conversion kits available with units which draw in air, which is heated and bubbled into the bath water.

There are many other sophisticated units available incorporating oxygen and the use of hot and warm water jets. These are professionally installed and the beauty therapist must be given instruction on their use. Remember the manufacturer is there to sell, so the beauty therapist must evolve appropriate safety and hygiene aspects when carrying out the treatment.

Thermal blanket

This blanket is specially designed and has insulating fabric padding and plastic sheeting covering the heating element. It measures approximately 5 ft 8 in by 4 ft 8 ins (1.72 m by 1.42 m), has a 'V' shape for the neck area and Velcro is used for fastening. There are two heat controls so the effect of the blanket can suit the client's tolerance level. It is useful for the home-visiting beauty therapist as it can fold away very easily.

There are virtually no contra-indications for its use and it is ideal to pre-heat the tissues for the older client with arthritic or rheumatic problems or for the younger client prone to sports injuries. The blanket requires about 10 minutes to heat up which gives the therapist enough time to prepare the couch with an ordinary blanket and a towel, and for the client to take a shower. Lay the thermal blanket on top of the towel and, for hygiene and protection, cover this with a large piece of plastic sheeting.

Settle the client comfortably on her back and wrap over the layer of plastic sheeting, then the thermal blanket using the velcro fastening to hold it in place and adjust the cut-out shape around the neck. Cover this with the ordinary blanket to ensure maximum heat is being retained.

Do not leave the client – the whole body is wrapped up like a parcel and when the warmth produces sweat, some clients feel trapped and at least want their arms outside the blankets. Talking to the client, and if necessary wiping the brow with a tissue or applying a cooling spray to the face, may help to alleviate this feeling. When the treatment has been completed, in about 20–30 minutes, remove the blanket and thermal blanket. Dispose of the plastic sheeting, advise the client to take a warm shower before proceeding with a manual massage or another treatment.

Remember to turn off the thermal blanket and remove the plug from its socket and, as soon as time permits, wipe the blanket with surgical spirit.

Apart from pre-heating the tissues, the thermal blanket can be useful after selected treatments. For instance, when certain essential oils or plant extracts in gels are used for specific purposes during massage, the heat from the blanket will assist their penetration.

Other methods

The infra-red lamp can also pre-heat the tissues and this has been described in Vol. 1, Chap. 31.

Paraffin wax baths can also be used as a relaxing heat bath and these are described in Chapter 14.

Chapter 10

Manual massage

Manual massage is a form of treatment which has been passed down through the centuries for thousands of years; for instance, a form of massage was certainly used by the Chinese in 3,000 BC. Generally, massage is described as manipulations of soft tissues of the body to stimulate the nervous and muscular systems and the local and general circulation of the blood and lymph. Therefore, its object is the restoration of function, and the re-establishment and re-shaping of the contours of the body.

One of the most important requirements for massage is a pair of good hands, strong and flexible, able to mould to every part of the body. Hand mobility exercises have been given in Vol. 1, Chap. 15 and these should be practised regularly. The standing position of the therapist is also important to avoid back strain by utilising body weight correctly, i e the feet should be placed in a position to allow the therapist to pivot freely from *walk standing* (which is one foot in front of the other) to *stride standing* (which is with both feet parallel and a few inches apart), with knees slightly flexed or, in some instances, bent. This enables the therapist to move rhythmically during massage and to use body weight effortlessly when needed. The massage couch (or plinth) should be at the correct working height and not too far away from the therapist to avoid stooping or stretching; it should also be wide enough to allow the client to turn over comfortably.

Classification of movements

Classification of movements are described in Vol. 1, Chap. 15, but are repeated here for easy reference, i.e. effleurage, petrissage, friction, tapotement and vibrations.

Effleurage or stroking

All stroking movements fall into this category. The palmar surface of one or both hands is laid flat on the part to be treated and with pressure applied over the skin in the direction of the venous or lymph flow (see Fig. 10.1 where effleurage is given to the leg). The hands must mould themselves to the contour of the body over which they are moving. Any degree of pressure may be applied from the lightest touch, superficial effleurage, to deep pressure, deep effleurage, dependent on the underlying structures. The hands should follow each other in slow and rhythmical movements without jerkiness or breaking contact with the skin. The cushions of the fingertips may by used but not the tips of the fingers as they cannot control the degree of pressure and the free edge of the nail could scratch the skin.

Care should be taken to ensure that the pressure of the strokes is very light over varicose veins and not at all if these are enlarged and also avoid any area where stretching of the skin could be harmful, i.e. newly-healed scar tissue.

The effects of effleurage are:

● venous circulation is improved;
● arterial circulation is aided by removal of congestion in the veins;
● lymphatic circulation is also improved with oxygen being brought to the area by the blood, and carbon dioxide and waste products being carried away;
● aids desquamation through an increase in sweat and sebum secretions;
● aids relaxation as the underlying muscles are nourished by an increase in blood supply and the fibres are loosened.

Petrissage

All pressure movements come under this heading and can be subdivided as follows.

Picking-up

The muscles are grasped with one hand, lifted away from the bone and relaxed and, as the muscles are released, the other hand grasps the area without breaking contact and lifts the muscles away from the bone in the opposite direction. The release must be sudden to be effective. Always ensure that the thumb is completely abducted and that the muscles are not pinched as this can cause pain. In the leg, for instance, the whole muscle is worked in this manner from origin to insertion, e.g. gastrocnemius. When the movement has been completed the hands slide back to the origin of the muscle to begin again. This movement can be used in conjunction with hacking for very heavy or fatty areas, i.e. gluteal region.

Kneading

There are various forms of kneading. It can be a single-handed movement whereby the heel of the hand is pressed on to the part and moved in small circles, not sliding the part but moving the tissues with it. Again the whole muscle is worked from origin to insertion, e.g. tibialis anterior.

Circular or palmar kneading is where the palms of the hands and fingers are used, care being exercised not to allow the heel of the hands to dig into the tissues. This type of kneading can be performed using one or both hands (double-handed kneading) working alternately on either side of the limbs (see Figs 10.2 and 10.3).

Finger kneading is a circular movement using the pads of the palmar surfaces of the thumb or first and second fingers, confining the massage to a small area. For instance, it is useful for breaking down nodules which are often found in the trapezius muscle.

Reinforced kneading (sometimes called 'ironing') uses both hands, one on top of the other, to obtain greater depth of pressure.

Squeezing

This movement is often used during kneading where the tissues are squeezed very gently (see Fig. 10.21).

Pincement

This type of massage is useful for fatty tissue. It is performed by lifting the superficial fascia between the fingers and the thumb and gentle squeezing or rolling with light but firm pressure. Care should be taken to ensure the skin is not pinched (see Fig. 10.5).

Skin rolling

This is very similar to the pincement movement but initially the hands are placed flat on an area and then the surface tissues are pulled or pushed away from the midline of the body to the sides. This is followed by the skin and tissues being picked up between fingers and thumbs and gently rolled backwards and forwards, again taking care not to pinch the skin (see Fig. 10.33).

Wringing

Wringing is to lift the tissues away from the bone and moving them (from side to side) across the length of the muscle, working the fingers of one hand with the thumb of the other hand. After the tissues have been stretched, the hands can move alternately along the muscles (see Fig. 10.14).

The effects of petrissage are:

- the compression and relaxation of muscle tissues causes the blood and lymphatic vessels to be filled and emptied. This increases the circulation and removal of waste products and so in turn eliminates fatigue;
- hard, contracted muscles are softened and relaxed;
- the skin, deep and superficial tissues are all stimulated to further activity;
- the sudden releasing of the stretched muscle fibres causes them to contract momentarily, so strengthening them;
- muscle tone is improved.

Friction

This is a small, deep circular or to-and-fro movement produced with the pads of the palmar surfaces of the first two fingers or thumb (see Figs 10.29 and

10.30). These are very localised movements and pressure must be completely released before moving on to another area. The skin and superficial structures must move together against the deeper structures to ensure that movement is not taking place on the skin surface.

The effects of friction are:

- breaks down fat and fibrous thickenings;
- removes oedema, i.e. swelling due to effusion of fluid into the tissues;
- stimulates circulation and brings fresh blood to the part;
- prevents the formation of skin adhesions and helps to loosen and stretch scar tissue.

Tapotement

This includes all percussion movements, which should be performed lightly and briskly to stimulate the tissues, but *never* applied over the abdominal cavity or the spinal column. These are subdivided as follows:

Hacking
This is performed with the elbows bent and the arms abducted; the hands should be at right angles to the wrists, with the palms facing each other but not touching. By a twist of the wrist, using the ulna side (dorsal surface) of the 5th, 4th and 3rd fingers loosely held, flick against the part being treated; first with one hand, then the other, in rapid succession. It is a light glancing movement – not a dull, heavy blow – and requires considerable practice to achieve the rhythm with both hands. Hacking is performed across the muscle fibres and should not be performed over bony areas, spastic muscles or painful conditions (see Fig. 10.6)

Clapping (or cupping)
This movement is used with the palms of the hands, slightly contracted, to form a hollow cup shape with the fingers closed (see Fig. 10.7). The whole of the cupped hand is lifted and dropped on the area to be treated, quickly followed by the other hand producing a rhythmical hollow, cupping sound. This movement is generally used on thighs and buttocks and over fatty tissue, and obviously cannot be used over bony areas.

Beating
Although similar to clapping it is a much heavier movement. A loosely clenched fist is used so that the dorsal part of the fingers and the heel of the hand strike the body. The arms are lifted to shoulder height and allowed to fall by their own weight, first one hand then the other, rhythmically and usually quite slowly. In beauty therapy it is only used over the gluteal region (see Fig. 10.24).

Pounding
This is another form of heavy percussion, similar to hacking in so far as the

stance of the beauty therapist is concerned, but the hands form a loosely clenched fist and the ulnar border of the hand strikes the part to be treated (see Fig. 10.25). The hands follow each other, turning inwards towards the therapist on the return of each stroke, resembling a circle. This movement is given over the buttocks and fleshy parts of the thighs and sometimes on the shoulders, but again cannot be used over bony areas.

The effects of tapotement are as follows:

Hacking
    causes muscle fibres to contract and so strengthens the muscle;
    given lightly for a short period of time, it causes contraction of the superficial vessels;
    given quite strongly for a longer period of time causes dilation of the vessels, erythema and change in skin temperature.

Clapping, beating and pounding
    locally produced erythema and rise in skin temperature;
● stimulates the nervous system, i.e. sensory nerves are irritated;
● softens adipose tissue;
● muscle activity is increased.

For most of these percussion movements the beauty therapist requires good posture with knees *bent* to avoid back strain.

Vibrations

Vibrations are a fine trembling movement performed with one or both hands using either the whole palmar surface or the pads of the fingertips and distal phalanx of the thumb. *Static* vibration is where the fingers are placed on a nerve and the muscles of the arm contract and relax rapidly to produce this fine trembling. When the vibrating fingers travel along the course of a nerve it is known as *running* vibrations. This can also be effected with the thumb and dorsal part of first finger, which can be seen in Fig. 10.36.

The effects of vibrations are:

    stimulates the nerves;
    relieves pain and fatigue;
    loosens scar tissue and stretches adhesions;
    fine vibrations have a sedative effect and can relax the client.

Contra-indications to massage

● over varicose ulcers or varicose veins which are bulbous;
    phlebitis or thrombosis;
    tumours or any unrecognisable lumps;
    in acute inflammatory conditions, i.e. around areas inflamed by boils or

carbuncles, bites or stings, acute joint conditions (rheumatoid arthritic
joints) swelling or bruising;
infectious skin diseases;
over recent scar tissue, allow time for internal healing;
when the temperature is raised;
any evidence of a spastic condition;
if the client has had a recent operation or fracture in the area.

As with all treatments, if the therapist has any concern about the health of
the client, medical advice should be sought.

There are occasions when common sense dictates the method of massage
or areas to be avoided when contra-indications are of a temporary nature.
For example, percussion movements would not be given to elderly or frail
clients. Abdominal massage would be omitted during menstrual flow or
during pregnancy; massage would not be given over painful areas, such as
clients who have taut, reddened skin due to over-exposure to the sun.

Preparation

The following should be ready, prior to the arrival of the client:

● the massage couch should be covered with a blanket or sheet, a large
  towel, a pillow and a length of paper tissue to cover these. The latter is
  usually a perforated couch roll, approximately 20 in (50 cm) in width;
  towels, large and small, should be folded at the foot of the couch;
● a trolley or table near the couch should contain roll pillows (or small
  towels made into a roll), head squares, massage medium (be it talcum
  powder, oil or cream), surgical spirit, a skin freshener, cotton wool and
  tissues;
  record cards should be to hand and completed at an appropriate time.

To prepare the client, assist with the removal of clothing and place them on a
nearby clothes hanger. It is very important to consider client modesty to
prevent any embarrassment between the therapist and the client. Many
female clients will take off all their clothes and lie naked on the couch; others
will prefer to keep on their bra and pants and their wishes must be respected.
Male clients (if being massaged by a female therapist) should wear their
briefs or a towel should cover the genitalia, again to prevent embarrassment.
In all probability the client will have come from a treatment which has preheated the tissues and will be more or less undressed and can lay supine on
the couch immediately and be wrapped up with towels and blanket. Interrup-
tions during a massage routine to change around towels can be minimised by
placing them correctly before covering up the client. Ensure that a small
towel (i.e. modesty towel) lies over the chest area and that a large towel is
arranged from the feet to the chest.

Sequence of massage

The following is a general sequence of massage which can be adapted once the therapist has gained confidence and skills. Although there are several schools of thought about the sequence, it is important to be methodical, performing the massage clockwise or anti-clockwise around the body. This will obviate the need to move frequently from one side of the couch to the other. The following routine is suggested:

right leg, including thigh; lower leg and foot; left leg (same as right leg); left arm (including hand); right arm (including hand); chest, abdomen, buttocks, back and shoulders.

The massage medium is normally chosen by the therapist but there are occasions when the client will request certain essential oils or creams; whichever medium is chosen it should be used sparingly and must be applied to the hands of the therapist first and *not* directly on to the client.

Ensure the client is comfortable, lying supine on the couch, pillow under the head and covered to keep warm. The therapist's hands should be washed and dried.

To commence the massage, uncover the client's right leg and apply the massage medium to the hands.

1. Effleurage from the tarsals (hands turned inwards, above each other) to cover the anterior surface of the limb to the femoral triangle; use superficial effleurage back to the tarsals and repeat (see Fig. 10.1).

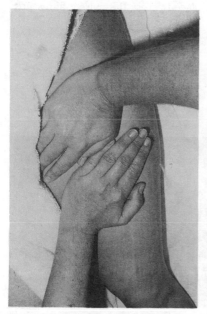

Fig. 10.1 Effleurage to the femoral triangle

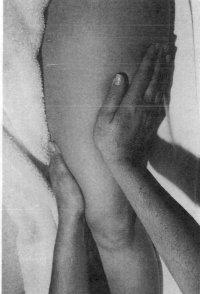

Fig. 10.2 Single-handed palmar kneading to the thigh, left hand supporting limb

The second stroke, or effleurage, will cover all the muscles on the lateral and medial sides of the leg, with the left hand following the gluteals but returning to the groin; again sliding hands back to the ankle, the movement is repeated.

The third stroke covers the posterior surface of the limb to the top of the leg where the hands curve into the groin, using slight pressure there, before returning to the achilles tendon to repeat the movement.

2. Slide hands to the insertion of the quadriceps (above the patella) and give single-handed palmar kneading over the vastus medialis and lateralis and rectus femoris from insertion to origin. The hand which is being used to knead will perform controlled circular movements and the free hand will support the thigh to prevent any rolling of the limb. Link these movements with effleurage (see Fig. 10.2).

3. Double-handed kneading follows until the entire anterior, medial and lateral surfaces of the thigh have been covered. Effleurage (see Fig. 10.3).

4. For the posterior surface of the thigh, raise the knee (supporting the foot with the therapist's thigh) and give alternative palmar kneading to the hamstring group of muscles. Start the movement at the widest part of the thigh and work down towards the popliteal space, always exerting forward pressure within the circular movements and return the hands with deep effleurage. This movement should be repeated three times (see Fig. 10.4).

5. Lower the leg and perform pincement movements to the thigh. The leg is rotated laterally and the hands are placed across the muscle fibres just

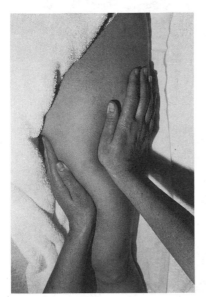

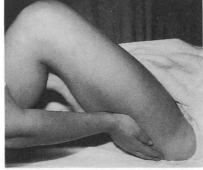

Fig. 10.3 Double-handed kneading to the thigh   **Fig. 10.4** Alternate palmar kneading to the posterior surface of the thigh

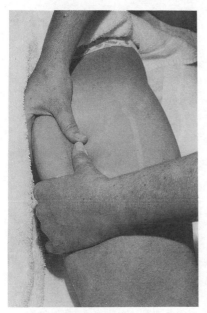

Fig. 10.5 Pincement to the thigh

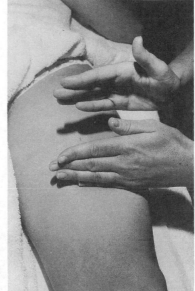

Fig. 10.6 Hacking

above the knee. The hands squeeze or roll out the tissues at the end of the stroke (see Fig. 10.5) and the hands return to start the movement again, working along the length of the muscle. This movement may require a knee support (i.e. a small pillow or rolled towel); it concludes with effleurage and the leg is then returned to its normal position.

6. Tapotements can be carried out on the thigh, i.e. hacking (see Fig. 10.6) and clapping (see Fig. 10.7), if this is considered to be beneficial, followed by effleurage from the knee to the groin.

7. Slide the hands down to the knee and effleurage with both hands around the knee joint finishing in the popliteal space. Follow this with deep finger kneading (see Fig. 10.8) and stroking (see Fig. 10.9) around the patella, i.e. first with digital stroking and then with the palmar surface of the hands.

8. To flex the leg slightly, place a support under the knee and perform the massage sequence for the lower leg and foot detailed in Vol. 1, Chap. 23, pp. 231–35 (figs 23.9 a–n). Effleurage the entire leg as given in 4.1 and finally cover the leg with the towel and blanket, leaving pillow or rolled towel under the knee as this will help client relaxation.

9. The therapist moves to the left side of the plinth, uncovers the left leg and repeats the massage sequence given for the right leg and foot. Ensure both legs are covered and warm.

10. Staying on the same side of the plinth, uncover the left arm. The arm is an awkward limb to massage and it is very helpful if the plinth is wide enough (or the client slim enough!) to allow the arm to rest upon it.

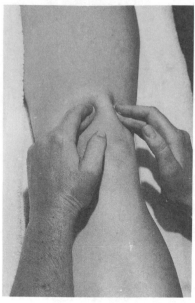

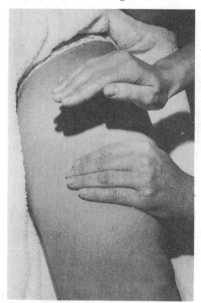

Fig. 10.7 Clapping

Fig. 10.8 Finger kneading around the patella

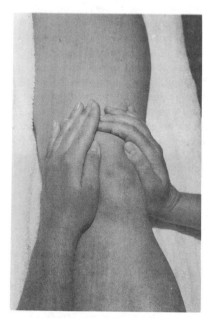

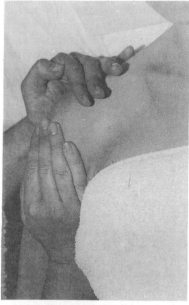

Fig. 10.9 Stroking around the patella

Fig. 10.10 Deep stroking over the shoulder joint

Effleurage can then be given to the entire arm with both hands starting at the palmar surface of the hand to the axilla (twice), followed by the lateral, medial and dorsal surfaces (twice). At the end of each effleurage there should be gentle pressure at the lymph glands. Often single-handed effleurage can be given instead, whereby the therapist holds the client's wrist and works from the wrist to the deltoid and axilla.

11. Deep stroking over the shoulder (about ten times) is given with alternate hands, i.e. with one hand commencing at the trapezius and the other at the deltoid, each hand finishing the stroke in the axillary glands at the back and front of the shoulder joint (see Fig. 10.10).

12. Palmar kneading movements are now given to the upper arm and fore-arm using alternate hands to support the arm, i.e. from the deltoid to the wrist covering the biceps and from the axilla to the wrist covering the triceps, linked with effleurage.

13. Alternate palmar kneading follows from the axilla to the wrist and, for support, it is useful to hold the hand of the client under the therapist's armpit (see Fig. 10.11). The hand is then placed on the couch to conclude the movement with both hands deep stroking to the shoulder.

14. Petrissage, consisting of picking up and wringing on the upper arm, follows. Using the right hand with the thumb well abducted, the muscles are grasped near their origin and lifted away from and carefully squeezed against the bone, relaxes them, while the left hand supports the limb (see Fig. 10.12). When this has been completed, wringing can begin on the

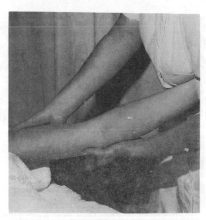

Fig. 10.11 Alternate palmar kneading to the upper arm

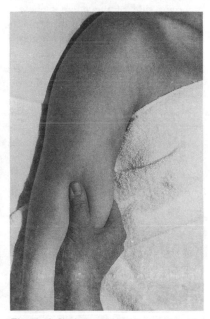

Fig. 10.12 Single-handed picking up of the biceps

deltoid, biceps and triceps, which involves grasping and lifting the tissues away from the bone and gently moving them from side to side i.e. a twisting effect, before moving on to another part.

15. Hacking (if this is considered beneficial) is performed with the client's arm bent at the elbow and placed across the chest. Effleurage the entire upper arm.

16. Perform the massage sequence for the forearm and hand as detailed in Vol. 1, Chap. 18, pp. 184–8 (Figs 18.10 – 18.21).

17. The therapist moves to the right hand side of the plinth and repeats steps 10–16 on the right arm and hand, reversing hand positions where necessary.

18. For the chest, the small towel may be taken down a little but should cover the nipples of the breast. Effleurage down the lateral sides of the neck into the supraclavicular glands, slide hands back to the neck and effleurage to the sternum, three times. On the last stroke fan the hands outwards across the pectoral muscles into the axilla and return to the sternum (see Fig. 10.13).

19. From the sternum, use deep stroking movements over the pectoral and deltoid muscles, the upper fibres of the trapezius muscle to the 7th cervical vertebra (twice), returning the hands back to the sternum. Repeat the same movement to the 5th vertebra (twice) and again to the occiput (twice). The elbows of the therapist should be bent and the head averted to prevent possible breathing in the face of the client.

20. From the sternum slide both hands to the pectoralis major muscle on the right side of the client's chest and perform picking up and wringing movements, concentrating on the muscle's insertion into the humerus (see Fig. 10.14). The movement is repeated to the left side of the chest, being linked with effleurage.

21. With reinforced hands use deep digital kneading over the left shoulder (see Fig. 10.15), covering the deltoid and upper fibres of the trapezius

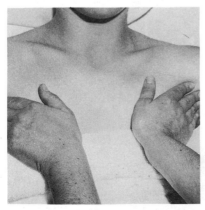

Fig. 10.13 Fanning hands outwards across pectoral muscles into the axillae

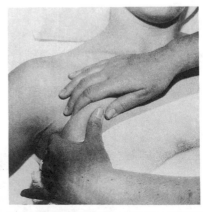

Fig. 10.14 Wringing of the pectoralis major muscle

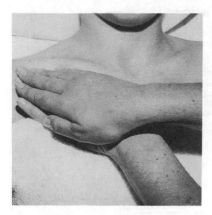

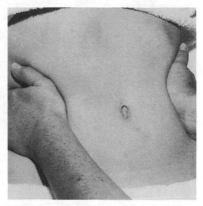

Fig. 10.15 Reinforced hands using digital kneading over the shoulder to the occiput

Fig. 10.16 Massage of the abdomen – hands using firm pressure returning to the symphysis pubis

muscle to the occiput and then move to the right shoulder to repeat the movement. Three times each side would be sufficient and it should be linked and completed with effleurage.

Finally the massage on the chest is completed by repeating the stroking movements over the pectoral and deltoid muscles as described in step 19.

22. To massage the abdomen, lift the small towel up to the neck, covering the breasts and shoulders, and ensure that the knees are supported by a pillow to relax the abdominal muscles. Deep stroking movements are used over the abdominal area which begins with both hands at the symphysis pubis and as they stroke upwards they divide and follow the iliac crests until the hands touch at the back, in the upper lumbar region. The hands return, using firm pressure from the back of the waist forwards and obliquely downwards to the symphysis pubis (see Fig. 10.16). It is a very slow movement and should be repeated at least three times.

23. Deep stroking to the upper abdomen follows with reinforced hands placed on the base of the sternum i.e. left hand over right hand. The hands move laterally to the right, over the ribs and return to the base of the sternum with firm pulling pressure over the upper abdomen (see Fig. 10.17). To repeat this to the left side of the body, apply the (reinforced) cushion tips of the fingers at the base of the sternum and slide them over the ribs; then push the hands upwards (see Fig. 10.18) over the upper abdomen, back to the sternum. This 'pulling' and 'pushing' movement is repeated four times on each side. It is difficult to perform unless the therapist has flexibility in the wrists and keeps the body weight evenly distributed, usually by stride standing with knees bent.

24. Deep kneading or stroking of the colon follows the direction of the flow of the contents of the digestive tract. Kneading is performed using a reinforced wrist with the hand cupped, and pressure being applied with the hypothenar eminence of the right hand. Starting at the right-hand side of the pelvis, work up the ascending colon, across the transverse

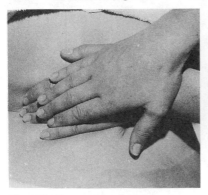

Fig. 10.17 Deep stroking of the upper abdomen with 'pulling' movement

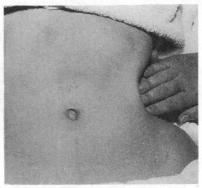

Fig. 10.18 Deep stroking of the upper abdomen with 'pushing' movement

colon and downwards over the area of the descending colon (see Fig. 10.19). This is linked with a light stroke over the lower rectus abdominis muscles back to repeat the kneading of the ascending colon etc. The movement is performed three times.

Deep digital stroking follows, i.e. with the fingers reinforced, again following the ascending, transverse and descending colon and is repeated three times (see Fig. 10.20).

If there is considerable adipose tissue present, kneading, wringing and picking up can be performed over the entire abdomen, otherwise squeezing should be confined to the lateral sides, at the tops of the hips and waist regions (see Fig. 10.21).

To complete the massage of the abdomen repeat the deep stroking movements detailed in step 22.

25. Remove the towels and help the client to turn over. Place the smaller towel over the shoulders and part of the back and the larger towel and blanket over the feet and legs with a pillow under the ankles to relieve

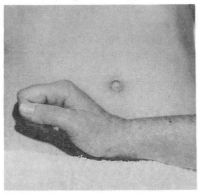

Fig. 10.19 Kneading of the colon

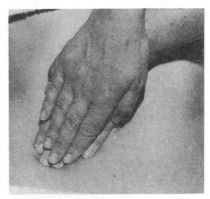

Fig. 10.20 Digital stroking of the colon

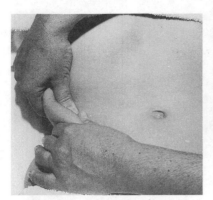

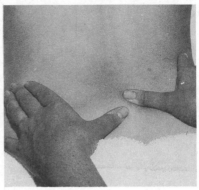

Fig. 10.21 Squeezing – the lateral sides of the abdomen

Fig. 10.22 Thumb frictions from the sacrum to coccyx

pressure of the toes on the plinth. Commence massage for the buttocks with deep effleurage movements from the lateral sides to the sacrum, being careful to avoid separation of the gluteal fold. Return to the sides with superficial strokes and repeat the movements firmly inwards and upwards six times.

26. Slide hands to the sacrum and make deep thumb frictions to the coccyx three times (see Fig. 10.22).
27. With reinforced hands give deep palmar kneading to the gluteal muscles on each side (see Fig. 10.23) three times followed by double-handed wringing, again three times each side and link with deep effleurage.
28. Tapotement movements follow, i.e. clapping, beating (see Fig. 10.24) pounding (see Fig. 10.25) and finally hacking, if these are considered to be beneficial. Repeat the deep effleurage given in step 25 and cover the buttocks with a towel to the sacrum, taking away the towel from the shoulders and back.
29. The back is probably the most important area for massage and the client

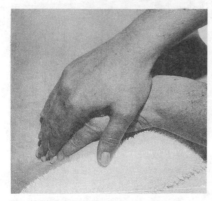

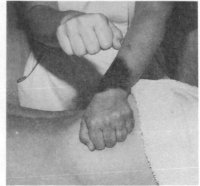

Fig. 10.23 Palmar kneading to the gluteals

Fig. 10.24 Beating

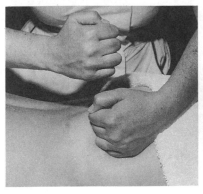

Fig. 10.25 Pounding

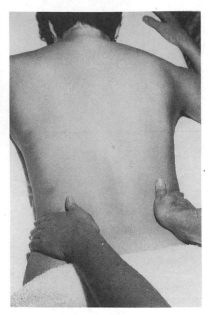

Fig. 10.26 Effleurage from sacrum to waist

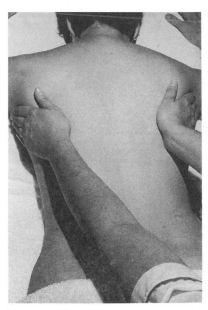

Fig. 10.27 Effleurage from sacrum to axillae

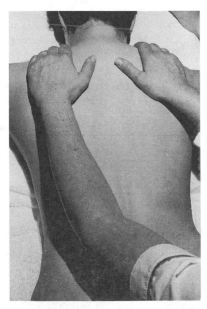

Fig. 10.28 Effleurage from sacrum to trapezius

should be made comfortable. The head can be placed to either side, but preferably a small towel should be put under the forehead or if the plinth has a 'breathing hole', split a tissue over this and let the client breathe through the hole.

Commence the massage with effleurage, upwards and outwards to the entire back. With the palmar surface of the hands perform two strokes from the sacrum to the waist level (see Fig. 10.26), i.e. external oblique muscles above the crests of ilium, two strokes to the axillae (see Fig. 10.27) and two strokes around the deltoid, over the trapezius muscles (see Fig. 10.28). The hands must return to the sacrum after each stroke.

Deep effleurage follows from the sacrum with the palmar surface of the hands following the erector spinae (i.e. either side of the spinous processes of the spine) to the occiput, using light effleurage to return to the sacrum. The second stroke takes the hands up the erector spinae, over the deltoid muscle and in towards the clavicle, returning to the sacrum. The third stroke follows the latissimus dorsi muscles to the axillary nodes, again returning to the sacrum.

30. Follow this with deep stroking to the scapula, where the thumbs are abducted and the hands stroke over the deltoid and trapezius muscles. The hands then draw the trapezius muscles back with the fingers while the thumbs stroke down both sides of the cervical vertebrae. This movement is repeated six times.

31. Deep thumb frictions are given to the trapezius and sternocleidomastoid muscles. This is better performed if the therapist leaves one hand on the client and moves to the head of the plinth. Slide the hands up towards the occiput and give deep finger frictions down the sides of the neck (see Fig. 10.29) and finger or thumb frictions along the upper fibres of the trapezius (see Fig. 10.30). This should be repeated at least three times.

32. Leaving one hand on the client, return to the side of the plinth and begin deep palmar kneading of the trapezius muscle, again first one side then

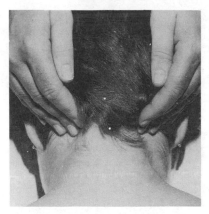

Fig. 10.29 Digital friction to sternocleidomastoid muscle

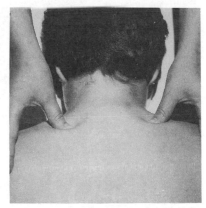

Fig. 10.30 Thumb friction to trapezius

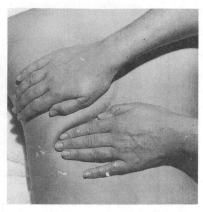

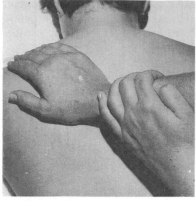

Fig. 10.31 Deep palmar kneading over back   **Fig. 10.32** Palmar kneading across the back

the other. If there is sufficient adipose tissue, wringing on the trapezius can follow. Intersperse these movements with effleurage especially if the areas becomes tender.

33. With reinforced hands, make deep palmar kneading movements over (right side of the body) the trapezius, teres major/minor, rhomboids, latissimus dorsi, external oblique muscles (see Fig. 10.31). Slide hands across the spine and continue kneading the same groups of muscles on the left side of the body and conclude with effleurage. Care must be taken to avoid any pressure on the spine.

34. Picking up and wringing movements follow (again, provided there is sufficient adipose tissue present). Cover the entire back smoothly and methodically, avoiding any breaks between one movement and another and linking them with effleurage.

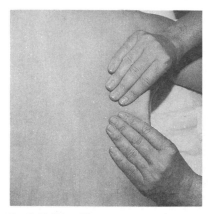

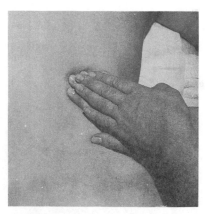

Fig. 10.33 Skin rolling   **Fig. 10.34** Deep digital kneading of the erector spinae

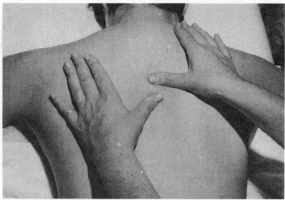

Fig. 10.35 Thumb friction on the spine

35. Use effleurage to the scapula and commence alternate palmar kneading over the entire back. This is where the hands make 'crossing' movements, using both forward and backward strokes firmly, so creating a kneading movement between the hands (see Fig. 10.32). On reaching the lumbar area, effleurage back to the scapula and repeat twice.

36. Slide the hands down to the axilla and perform skin rolling on both sides of the back, i.e. rolling the tissues towards the spine smoothly down the back until the side nearest the therapist has been completed but rolling the tissues away from the spine on the side furthest away from the therapist (see Fig. 10.33). Link these movements with effleurage.

37. Deep kneading on the erector spinae follows, either with a reinforced wrist with the hand cupped and pressure being applied with the hypothenar eminence of the hand, or deep digital kneading, as seen in Fig. 10.34. This is performed once on each side of the spine, returning to the occiput with effleurage.

38. Thumb frictions are applied to the spine but care should be taken to avoid pressure on the bony vertebrae as this can cause discomfort (see Fig. 10.35). Use slow effleurage on the erector spinae to return the hands to the occiput and repeat the movement three times.

39. Finger kneading is then applied down the erector spinae to the sacrum, followed by deep thumb kneading over the sacrum. The palmar surface of the hand is used to effleurage the sacral area.

40. Hacking and clapping can be applied if this is thought to be beneficial. Commence with very light hacking over the cervical area, changing to heavier hacking down the thoracic and lumbar areas where adipose tissue is present. It is important to work very methodically over the whole of the back, but being careful not to use tapotements on the spine. Clapping follows where fatty tissue is evident. All the movements are linked with effleurage.

41. Vibrations are given from the sacrum to the erector spinae to the occiput returning to the sacrum with effleurage (see Fig. 10.36).

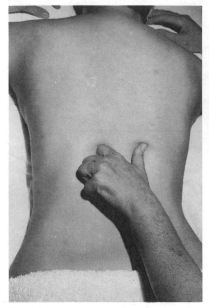

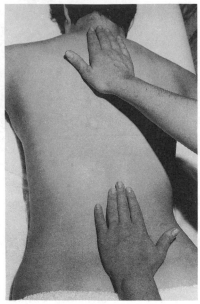

Fig. 10.36 Vibrations to the erector spine

Fig. 10.37 Alternate palmar stroking down the length of the spine

42. From the sacrum, slow deep strokes are given to the entire back, as given in step 29 but finishing at the occiput.
43. To conclude the massage, alternate palmar stroking is used down the length of the spine. One hand is placed flat on the cervical region and is stroked slowly down the spine and as it reaches the sacrum, the other hand is placed on the cervical region to commence the same stroke (see Fig. 10.37). These movements are repeated six times but each stroke becomes lighter until the last stroke is 'feather-like', finishing at the sacrum with slight pressure.

After the massage has been completed the client may return to the supine position and left to rest, covered with towels and blanket to keep warm. Finally, assist the client to a sitting position (to regain equilibrium) and remove blanket and towels. If oil has been used, any excess may be removed with an astringent or hot towels. Assistance should be given to replace gown or clothing. After the client has left the cubicle, the couch must be stripped of paper, and towels placed in laundry basket.

Chapter 11

Mechanical massage

The value of massage being performed by mechanical means lies in the increased depth effect, which is often difficult to achieve with the hands alone.

Gyratory vibrators

A gyratory vibrator is a heavy-duty vibrator used for general body work. It is normally a floor-standing unit, with the weight of its motors on a pedestal supported by four legs. From the motor a flexible drive-shaft extends to a gyratory head to which an applicator head is attached. There is a range of applicator heads, made from foam or rubber and/or polyurethane, and these are used for specific purposes, for example:

- a foam or soft rubber head has a similar effect to that of effleurage;
- a hard rubber head has an effect similar to that of petrissage; and
- a spiked head is used to increase superficial blood and lymph circulation and has a similar effect to that of tapotement.

Several types of applicator heads are shown in Fig. 11.1.

Gyratory vibrators operate in a circular movement and, by varying the pressure, position and type of applicator head, the therapist is able to control the depth of penetration of the vibrations.

There are also available hand-held versions of heavy-duty vibrators which produce similar effects, but because of the weight these are more tiring for the therapist to use. They have a two-speed control on the handle, the slow speed for deep penetration and the fast speed to stimulate circulation. Various applicator heads are available, similar to those supplied with the floor-standing unit. It should be noted that these hand-held models have a powerful motor enclosed in a small area and despite small circulating fans built into the mechanism, they are inclined to get warm during use. It is not advisable to continuously run these machines for more than 15 minutes as they will become hot, and damage will be caused to their insulation.

The effects of vibratory massage

- Helps to soften hard fatty deposits and is therefore useful for spot reduction.

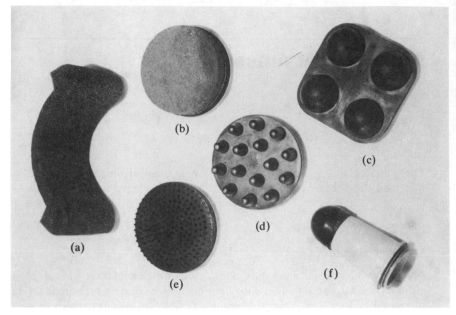

Fig. 11.1 Types of applicator heads for vibratory massage

(a) 'horse-shoe' head for arms and legs
(b) soft head for stroking movements
(c) hard heads for petrissage
(d) knobbly head for tapotment
(e) spiking head for tapotment
(f) cone head applicator for nodules and small areas

● Increases blood circulation and lymphatic flow.
● Relieves tension by relaxing muscle fibres.
● Relieves aches and pains.
● Aids desquamation.
● Improves cellular activity and therefore improves skin tone.

Contra-indications to gyratory massage

● All those listed for manual massage.
● Over the abdomen or on the breasts. Here there is lack of bony support and, because of the power of these machines, there is the risk of damage to these sensitive areas. However, it is appreciated that there is a school of thought that the small cone applicator head can be used up the ascending, across the transverse, and down the ascending colon, but it is difficult to be aware of the depth of pressure. It is safer for these areas to be massaged by hand.
● Thin or elderly clients with a lack of subcutaneous tissue.
● Extremely hairy areas (do not use applicators that could pull hairs and cause discomfort).

- Bony areas.
- Around or over any metal plates in the body.

Preparation

This is the same as for manual massage (see Chapter 10). Ensure that the record card has been completed before commencing the treatment. As this type of massage lacks sensitivity and can be rather impersonal, some manual massage movements should be included to maintain a personal contact by the therapist's hands.

To aid relaxation of the muscles some pre-heating of the tissues is useful, preferably infra-red or sunbed which does not cause the body to sweat for any length of time. Talcum powder is always used for a vibratory massage to ensure the smooth movement of the applicator heads and this is not always possible if the client is sweating after the use of the steam cabinet or sauna. Another reason for using powder and not oil is that the latter causes soiling and damage to the applicators, i.e. rubber to perish.

The powder should always be applied to the hands of the therapist and not directly onto the client. The various applicator heads are chosen for different parts of the body and for either a relaxing or stimulating massage. Stopping the massage to change heads unnecessarily can be irritating to the client and therefore it is important initially to assess the type of treatment to be given and decide when and how often to change the applicator head.

Sequence of massage

Ensure that the client is comfortable, lying supine on the couch, pillow under the head and covered to keep warm. The therapist's hands should be washed and dried. To commence the massage, uncover the client's legs and apply the powder to the hands.

1. Effleurage both legs with the hands. Take the vibrator in one hand and with a smooth applicator head attached (i.e. sponge or rubber), apply long, sweeping, upward strokes in the direction of the venous and lymphatic flow, to the front and sides of the legs to the inguinal glands. Always use the free hand to maintain contact with the client, especially when the vibrator finishes one stroke to commence another. Repeat the sequence to the other leg.
2. Depending upon the adipose tissue present and the size of the thighs, the applicator head may be changed to a ball-studded type (or knobbly head). It is used in a circular upward movement, with the free hand of the therapist providing support and resistance to the strokes, and again maintaining contact with the skin.
3. The applicator head needs to be changed again and talcum powder applied to continue up the body. The abdomen can be massaged manually. Cover the areas already massaged and move to the chest and use the appropriate applicator head to perform stroking movements from the upper sternum to the axillae, following the lymph flow.

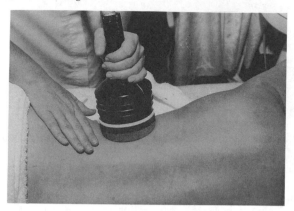

Fig. 11.2 Vibratory massage using 'soft' head on the back

4. Follow this with stroking movements on the upper arms and, to avoid changing heads, any rough skin or excess adispose tissue over the biceps or triceps muscles can be dealt with when the client is lying prone.
5. Request the client to turn over and apply talcum powder from the ankles to the cervical area. For a relaxing massage simply use the applicator with the foam or soft rubber head and commence slow sweeping movements over the entire body, always in the direction of the venous flow with the free hand maintaining contact with the body (see Fig. 11.2).
6. For a stimulating massage or a figure correction treatment, i.e. thighs and buttocks, cover the shoulders and concentrate on this area. Choose

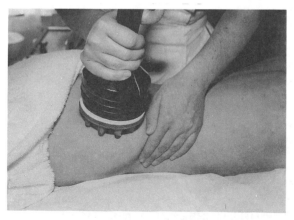

Fig. 11.3 Vibratory massage using 'knobbly' head to the buttocks

an appropriate applicator for the type of fat or adispose tissue present, usually a ball-studded or knobbly head and massage from just above the popliteal space along the medial, lateral and posterior muscles of the thigh. Work across the muscle fibres, using the supporting hand to push the muscles towards the applicator head (see Fig. 11.3) and finish with manual effleurage. Repeat for the other leg. With the same applicator head, move on to the buttocks.

Perform stroking movements followed by deep pressure movements, always working inward to the gluteal fold and again using the supporting hand to push the muscles towards the applicator head. Cover these areas with a towel.

7. It may be necessary to change the applicator head for the waist to effect a wringing movement without discomfort – this again depends on the amount of fat present.

8. Remove the towel from the shoulders and use the appropriate applicator for the upper arms.

9. Change to a cone-shaped applicator head and very slowly work along the trapezius and down the erector spinae, being careful to avoid the spinous processes of the vertebrae. This will relax and ease tense muscles.

10. Finally, use a foam or soft rubber applicator head to work all over the body in the direction of the lymphatic flow and this will completely relax the client. The personal contact with the client is maintained by finishing the treatment with alternate palmar stroking down the length of the spine as detailed in Chap. 10, step 43, Figure 10.37.

Switch off the appliance, remove the plug from its socket, tidy the leads and put away.

As with a manual massage; the client may return to the supine position and be left to rest covered with towels and blanket to keep warm and later assisted to a sitting position and helped with gown or clothing. After the client has left the cubicle or salon, the couch should be made ready for the next client.

Maintenance of the equipment

The applicator heads should be cleaned after use by washing them with tepid water, a mild soap and a diluted antiseptic, i.e. TCP, Dettol or Savlon (but not with surgical spirit), then rinsed and dried thoroughly. If the vibrator is in constant use, two or three sets of applicator heads will be required to ensure that the heads are always clean and dry. Always replace the heads as they become worn to avoid any discomfort to the client.

The machine should be freed from talc between treatments and thoroughly cleaned at the end of the day. As with all electrical appliances, regular servicing is important.

Vibratory massage using essential oils

This is a vibratory machine which can emit a mist of essential oils through the

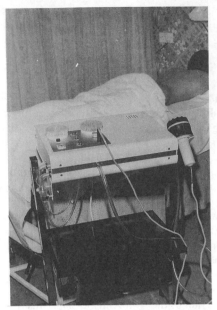

Fig. 11.4 Vibratory machine used for essential oils

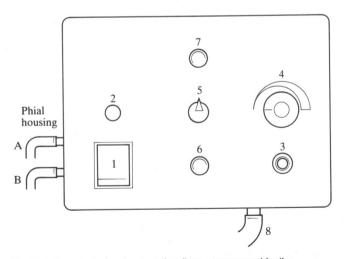

Fig. 11.5 Control panel and features for vibratory massage with oils
1. mains on/off switch (amber glow for 'on');
2. external fuse housing (1.6A rating);
3. cable socket for massage head pin attachment;
4. intensity or speed control. Minimum–maximum as indicated;
5. selector switch for phials
6. amber light will indicate when selector switch is downward and phial 'B' activated;
7. amber light will indicate when selector switch is upward and phial 'A' activates;
8. fitting point for plastic sleeve attachment running from the massage head to unit.

applicator heads during the massage. Fig. 11.4 shows the machine and Fig. 11.5 gives details of the controls. The unit has the main rubber applicator head and large brush heads and at the side of the unit there are two glass phials for the essential oils. By operating the selector switch a pump will atomize an oil to produce the mist which passes through the massage heads by means of minute air ducts. By having two phials it means that the therapist can select two products and switch from one to the other during the treatment. The products used in the phials must not be water-based, i.e. tonic water or toners.

Contra-indications and preparation are the same as for the gyratory massage detailed above, pp. 238–239. The massage sequence is also similar when using the rubber head, i.e. following the direction of the venous and lymphatic flow. The use of the brush heads effects a very stimulating brush massage and can be used in conjunction with appropriate skin peeling products to cleanse the skin prior to massage or to any other suitable body treatment. The speed of the massage is adjusted by the intensity control.

Maintenance of equipment

The rubber head can be cleaned with soapy water and alcohol. The brush heads, which are made of bristle and nylon, may discolour (depending on the product used) but this is not important so long as they are cleaned thoroughly and allowed to dry naturally. Care must be exercised with the glass phials and these should be washed with hot, soapy water and dried well before further use.

Audio-sonic vibrators

Audio-sonic vibrators work on a very different principle from mechanical vibrators as they produce sound waves in surface body tissue to encourage circulation of the blood and lymph and relieve tension. The depth of penetration beneath the skin is up to about 2 in (5 cm) in soft tissue and are therefore not recommended for use over bony areas. However, they can be used on areas of tension or hyper-sensitivity without discomfort, i.e. fibrositis found in the muscle sheaths of the back. The deep penetration of audio-sonic vibrators makes it useful in the treatment of soft fat, i.e. 'cellulite' conditions and adipose deposits in sensitive areas, where the gyratory vibrator would be contra-indicated. These vibrators are small and come in a hand-held form and are only suitable for localised areas of the body, but nevertheless can be very effective.

In the main, the applicator heads for the audio-sonic vibrators are made of hard plastic; a smooth disc-shaped head, about an inch in diameter which is used for general work and a small rounded ball-shaped head which is used for concentration in small areas, i.e. between muscle fibres or around joints. On the head of the vibrator is a control knob, which controls the current to the motor, and by turning this, the level of intensity is increased or decreased. The frequency is 50–100 Hz. Beneath the head of the vibrator lies a plate into which the applicator head is attached and in the handle of the vibrator is the on/off switch.

The effects of audio-sonic vibratory treatments

Causes compression and rarefaction in the tissue.
Relieves tension in muscle fibres.
Relieves aches and pains.
Improves blood and lymph flow.

Contra-indications to audio-sonic vibratory treatments

Bony areas.
Inflammation of the skin, i.e. sepsis.
Over the abdomen.
Very thin clients.

Preparation

Preparation is the same for any other massage, always ensuring that the areas not being treated are kept covered and warm. Any massage medium may be used (the plastic head is impervious to oil).

Sequence of massage

The audio-sonic vibrator can be applied to the body as a whole in a similar manner to the gyratory vibrator, but normally it is confined to specific areas. It is often used during a manual or gyratory massage for sensitive regions, e.g.

Fibrositis nodules in the trapezius muscle can often be broken down by stroking along the length of the muscle, from insertion to origin. This can be followed by increasing the level of intensity and using circular movements over the same muscle (see Fig. 11.6). Care must be taken when altering the frequency to ensure the correct depth of vibration.

Migraine-type headache can be relieved by stroking the upper fibres of the trapezius muscle to the occiput, using a mild frequency.

Soft fat deposits on the inside of the thighs can be rarefied by stroking the length of the adductor muscles. These deposits can also be found on the medial side of the patella and the vibrator can be used on the sartorius and vastus medialis muscles to good effect.

● Soft fat deposits on the triceps of the upper arms are also areas which can be sensitive and the use of the audio-sonic vibrator is also useful here.

Again this is a mechanical massage and, as only one hand is required to

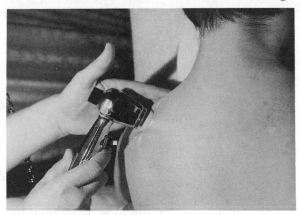

Fig. 11.6 Audio-sonic over the trapezius muscle

operate the vibrator, the free hand should remain on the body to maintain personal contact.

As with all electrical appliances, switch off, remove the plug from its socket, tidy the lead but before putting the vibrator away the applicator head should be removed for washing clean.

Underwater massage

This massage is performed in a hydrotherapy bath as shown in Fig. 11.7. This type of massage should not be confused with the underwater massage given by a physiotherapist, whereby a client is immersed in the water, usually supported by a sling, and massage is given with the physiotherapist standing in the water.

To install the bath, hot and cold water connections, drainage and an electrical supply will be required.

As will be seen, the bath has various controls and these should be well understood to ensure a smooth, controlled and comfortable treatment.

To fill the bath, open tap No. 2 for warm water and tap No. 3 for cold water (the spout is No. 10 on the diagram) until the water is about 2–3 in (5–8 cm) *above the level of the suction sieve*, which is marked as No. 11. This is very important as the bath is supplied with a special pump, operated when switch No. 5 is activated, and if there is no water in the bath, or the level of the water is below the suction sieve, the pump will be damaged.

Check the temperature of the water which should be approximately 35–38°C (95–100°F) and this is registered by the thermometer control, marked in the diagram as No. 8.

The pressure of the water jet is dependent upon:

● the position of the switch (No. 6) whereby, when completely open, the pressure will be at its highest, i.e. it will circulate maximum water volume; and

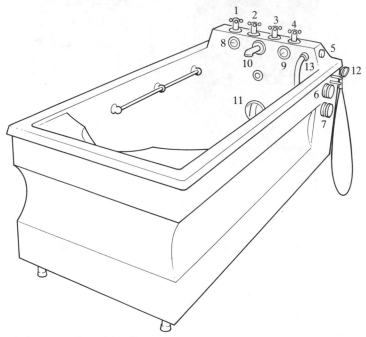

1. hot water through handles;
2. warm water to fill bath;
3. cold water to fill bath;
4. water cooling system;
5. on/off switch;
6. pressure switch and regulator;
7. whirlpool bath;
8. thermometer;
9. manometer;
10. bath inlet/spout;
11. suction sieve;
12. hand shower, warm-cold;
13. hose to which nozzle is attached.

Fig. 11.7 Hydro-therapy bath for underwater massage

● the type of nozzle attached to the hose (No. 13), i.e. the nozzle with a small opening will have a high pressure but a smaller water volume, whereas the nozzle with a larger opening will have a lower pressure but a higher water volume.

The pressure of the water jet, as it leaves the nozzle, is being registered by the manometer, which is marked on the diagram as No. 9.

Both the manometer and the thermostat should be watched carefully when giving an underwater massage. If there is a need for the water temperature to be decreased, the tap marked on the diagram as No. 4 can be opened and the water will enter the bath from the jets in the handles fixed just inside the top of the bath. However, if the water temperature needs to be increased the tap marked No. 1 on the diagram can be opened and the hot water will enter the bath through the suction sieve (No. 11). This refinement obviates the need to use the warm and cold water taps (No. 2 and 3) with water pouring from the spout (No. 10).

On the diagram, switch No. 7 is only used for the built-in whirlpool jets and should be kept closed during an underwater massage.

Finally, the hand shower, which is shown as No. 12 on the diagram, is self-explanatory.

The effects of the underwater massage

● Increases circulation of blood and lymph flow.
● Breaks down hard adipose tissues.
● Relieves tension by relaxing muscle fibres.
● Useful for spot reduction.

Contra-indications to underwater massage

● All those listed for both manual and vibratory massage.
● Any client who may bruise easily.
● Any client who has a fear of water, or who has a tendency to faint when the body becomes slightly over-heated.

Preparation

Prior to the arrival of the client, the bath should be run and the temperature checked. This is a very deep massage and can be tiring; therefore ensure that the record card has been completed prior to the commencement of the treatment. For a masseur, most female clients prefer to wear a bikini or swimsuit, and for the masseuse, male clients are requested to wear swimming trunks or briefs.

The client should be assisted with the removal of clothing, requested to shower (if this is considered necessary), and a shower cap be given for the client to wear in the bath (or the hair tied back). The bath is quite tall and it is normal to provide steps. For hygiene purposes these must be covered with a clean towel for each client.

Sequence of massage

Assist the client into the bath and allow time for relaxation in the warm water for about three minutes with the head supported by the rubber head rest provided. During this time select and attach the nozzle to the hose.

1. Hold the hose firmly and direct the nozzle downwards into the bath and switch on the pump (switch No. 5). Adjust the pressure of the water by opening or closing the switch (No. 6). As the water jet moves over the body, indentations will be observed and you should ensure that these are not too deep, otherwise bruising will occur (see Fig. 11.8).

2. Commence with massage between the metatarsals and, as the feet are usually quite thin, the water jet pressure should be low. Take the jet up the lateral and medial sides of the leg towards the knee, being careful to avoid the tibia.

3. Make strokes around the patella and continue up the thigh. Depending on the amount of adipose tissue present, check the pressure of the water and make three strokes on the lateral side to the waist, being careful to avoid bony areas, i.e. crest of ilium, and then to the anterior and medial aspect of the thigh. It is useful here to support the thigh by placing the free hand on the popliteal space.

4. Repeat steps 2 and 3 for the other leg.

5. Take one arm and massage from the metacarpals to the elbow joint and from there to the axilla, covering lateral, anterior and medial sides of the arm. Repeat for the other arm.

6. Turn the client over, move the head strap to provide a support for the chin. Massage the posterior side of the leg, avoiding the popliteal space, to the beginning of the buttocks. Repeat for the other leg.

7. For the buttocks, massage from the lateral side and stroke towards the gluteal fold, covering the gluteal maximus and medius and repeat for the other side.

8. The client should then turn on to the back and raise the knees to ensure that the back and shoulders are under the water. For support the client can hold onto the internal handles. Take the water jet from the gluteus medius over all the muscles of the back and shoulders, i.e. oblique external, erector spinae, latissimus dorsi, trapezius and deltoid, being careful

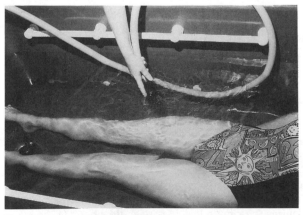

Fig. 11.8 Underwater massage to the leg

to avoid the spinous processes of the vertebrae. This should be carried out, first one side of the back and then the other.

During the treatment closely watch the temperature of the water.

N.B. There is another method to perform massage of the buttocks and back to replace steps 6, 7 and 8. Lower the head strap and turn the client to one side with the back facing the therapist and again, shoulders and back under the water. Take the water jet from the gluteus maximus and massage all the muscles of the back and finish at the trapezius and deltoid. The number of strokes performed will depend on the size of the client. The client should turn to the other side, and the therapist moves to the opposite side of the bath and completes the massage of the back and shoulders.

9. Turn off the water pressure and allow the client to rest on the back and relax for a few minutes. The hand shower may now be used if required. The client should be assisted out of the bath, wrapped in towels and taken to an area to rest for 15 minutes before dressing.

Maintenance of equipment

Remove the plug and allow the bath water to drain away. With a diluted antiseptic, wash the interior and the head rest, then take the hand shower to rinse out the bath and dry well. Place all used towels into the laundry basket.

Maintenance is minimal, providing all the nozzles and water outlets are kept clean and the pump is never used without the water level being above the suction sieve. Ensure regular servicing.

Intermittent compression massage.

This is a treatment which is helpful in improving venous and lymphatic circulation of the limbs using inflatable leggings, known as 'boots' and arm sleeves. The machine itself is an electrically operated pump used for inflation and the smaller units, suitable for beauty therapy, have indicator lights for on/off switch and for air pressure and an air-pressure gauge or controller. At the side of the machine are outlets into which are pushed the long plastic tubes from either the boots, or the arm sleeves. As the arm sleeves are rarely required the use of the boots are explained here. These come in various sizes, i.e. large, medium, and half leg, and are made of washable polyurethane material and all are fitted with zips to facilitate ease of use. At the top of the boot is an outlet with a ring which is pulled out to deflate the boots.

The effects of intermittent compression massage

● Improves venous flow and can be used over varicose veins at low pressure.

Helps to eliminate waste toxins.
Improves both peripheral and lymphatic oedema.
● Useful for sports injuries, where bruising or oedema is evident.
relieves feeling of tired, heavy or swollen legs and ankles.

There are many other uses for this treatment in the hands of specialists but outside the scope of beauty therapy.

Contra-indications

Acute thrombo-phlebitis.
Any known or suspected recent deep vein thrombosis.
Acute pulmonary oedema.
Congestive heart failure.

Preparation

Ensure that the client's record card has been completed, especially any medical history, before commencing the treatment. Place the machine on a stable surface, plug into a socket and switch on. Both indicator lights will illuminate and the unit should be left for approximately 5–10 minutes to achieve normal running pressure, during which time the client should remove shoes, tights/stockings etc., and lie on the couch in a semi-reclining position.

Method of use

The legs should be covered with gauze or similar material to prevent excess-

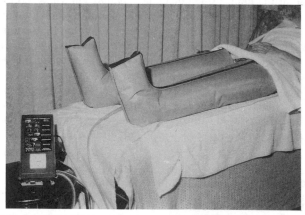

Fig. 11.9 Intermittent compression massage using the 'boots'

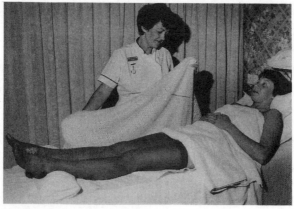

Fig. 11.10 Cool stocking treatment

ive perspiration. There are also various creams or gels available which can be massaged into the legs and then covered with plastic sheeting.

The client puts her legs into the boots and these are zipped up. The long plastic tubes are fitted into the outlets at the side of the machine and the pull ring is inserted into the valve. The air-pressure control, which will read from 20 to 120 mm Hg, should be turned slowly and the treatment commenced at approximately 25 mm Hg. The client will feel inflation and decompression of the tissues on alternate legs and the therapist should adjust the pressure accordingly to ensure that the compression is adequate but not too strong for a comfortable treatment (see Fig. 11.9).

When the treatment has been completed, usually after 30 minutes, the pull ring is released to allow for deflation before unzipping the boots. Use damp cotton wool to remove perspiration, creams or gels from the legs and pat dry with a tissue.

There is an optional therapy which can be applied, namely a cool stocking treatment, ideal for tired or swollen legs. This comprises a pair of high-denier stockings which are rolled and soaked in a specialised solution and put on the legs. The ankles are placed on a pillow to raise and rest the legs. The client will feel an immediate fresh cooling sensation. Local temperature is reduced, causing blood vessels to contract; circulation is improved so that any stagnant venous blood is returned more freely towards the heart. Swelling is reduced and with regular treatment unsightly veins (not varicose veins) are diminished. The client may feel quite cold and a blanket should be at hand to ensure comfort (see Fig. 11.10).

The stockings are removed and thoroughly washed and can be used for more treatments on the same client, or given to the client for home use. The usual courtesies are extended to the client before leaving the salon.

The maintenance of the equipment is minimal. The plastic tubes must be kept clean and the boots washed (inside and outside) after use.

Chapter 12

Vacuum suction

Vacuum (or suction) massage is an electrical method for lymphatic drainage. It is also an extremely effective spot reducing treatment for parts of the body prone to fatty deposits, i.e. hips, thighs and upper arms, which are difficult to slim down by exercise or manual massage.

The vacuum suction machine has a control panel with an on/off switch, an intensity control, a light and a pressure gauge which registers the intensity of the vacuum. There are clear perspex cups of varying sizes which are attached at one end to flexible plastic tube/s, the latter being connected to the machine.

The unit has a motor with a rotary pump which draws in air from the cups applied to the skin. This causes the skin under the cups to be pushed into the cup space in an attempt to replace the air that the pump has removed. There is an outlet, usually at the back of the unit, which vents the air into the atmosphere. Ensure that the mains electrical current is AC 220/240 volts.

There are two methods of vacuum suction, i.e. static and 'gliding'. For static vacuum suction the cup is left in one position and the inverse pressure effect causes the tissues to rise up in the cup to produce erythema and vascular interchange in the area. The suction is broken by placing a finger under the rim of the cup and it is moved to another position. If several cups are used, these are moved around alternately. Due to the pressure, pulsations can break down fatty deposits but the gliding method of vacuum suction will assist the removal of waste products along the lymphatic vessels to the lymphatic system (see Chapter 4). This involves the drawing up of the tissue in a single cup and moving it in the direction of the lymphatic flow to the nearest lymph node.

The effects of vacuum suction massage

- Increases blood and lymph flow.
- Produces erythema, thereby improving blood supply to the area.
- Improves local absorption of adispose deposits.
- Reduces oedema caused by trauma, i.e. a sprained ankle, bursitis or synovitis.
- Helps prevent chilblains.

However, if vacuum suction is used for spot reduction (i.e. to remove fat from unwanted areas), the client should undertake and maintain a healthy slimming diet. It is also important to appreciate that this is a cumulative treatment. A course of 10 or 12 treatments, twice weekly, should be recommended and results can be realised after the 6th treatment.

Contra-indications to vacuum suction

Cardio-vascular conditions i.e. thrombosis, phlebitis, etc.;

oedema of organic origin, i.e. swelling caused by kidney or cardio vascular problems;

over varicose veins;

● during pregnancy or immediately after childbirth (allow at least three months to elapse);

avoid the breasts as the area is too sensitive;

● avoid the abdomen during menstruation;

● avoid the abdomen if the client is prone to hernia;

skin diseases or near parts affected by inflammation, other than chilblains;

● avoid skin abrasions, sunburn and bruises;

over or near scar tissue (for a very small scar leave for at least six months and for a larger scar i.e. hysterectomy, avoid for at least two years);

● crêpey or ageing skin or dilated capillaries.

Preparation

The following is suggested for the 'gliding' application as this is generally accepted as the usual form of treatment.

Have ready on the table/trolley a suitable thin, oil liquid, i.e. glycerine. Thicker oils (olive, corn, sunflower or castor oils) tend to become sticky with constant use of the cup over the skin and the efficiency of the treatment is reduced. At the end of the treatment cologne or a tonic or talcum powder will be used and these should be to hand. Ensure that the machine is plugged in, the tubing is pushed directly on to the outlet, there are no cracks in the cups and the dial is at zero.

On arrival of the client, check for any contra-indications and, if a course of treatments is advised for spot reduction, take measurements of the area concerned. At this time, the therapist can decide on the size of the cup/s to be used, as these should always be smaller than the area being treated to prevent any leakage of air at the edges of the cup/s. For guidance, the following is suggested:

small limbs or small areas of fat, a cup of 1 in (2.5 cm) in diameter;
a fairly thick thigh, a cup of 2 in (5 cm) diameter;

- a very thick or fat thigh, a cup of 3 in (7.5 cm) diameter;
- buttocks, which are fat, a cup of 4 in (10 cm) in diameter.

The intensity of the treatment is decided by the vacuum produced and this is obtained by placing a finger or thumb over the hole in the centre of the cup, turning the intensity control (which provides a controlled leak of air into the system) to the predetermined vacuum required. See Table 12.1 for suggested

Table 12.1   Initial vacuum requirements

The area	Initial vacuum percentage
Thighs – medial	7
–anterior and lateral	8
Buttocks	8
Abdomen and midriff	6–7
Back and shoulders	8
Legs – anterior	8
– posterior	7
Arms – anterior	6
– posterior	7

The percentage should be lowered by 1% vacuum for older clients.

initial vacuum required for the various parts of the body, but with experience the therapist will increase or decrease the amount of vacuum required for specific areas or conditions. Vacuum suction is best used on hard or trapped fat as its use on soft fat could cause stretch marks if the therapist is not extremely careful.

Sequence of massage

Some form of pre-heating the tissues is beneficial to warm through the subcutaneous tissue and relax the muscles. The client should lie on the couch in a comfortable position and be kept warm, i.e. any areas not being treated should be well covered. It is normal to treat only one area at a time; therefore the sequence of the massage will be given for each part. In general terms, each area should be covered with a thin film of oil and the cup chosen in the operating hand.

When the cup is placed on the skin the tissue will rise into the cup and the little finger or the tip of the index finger should be brought under the cup to release the vacuum at the end of each stroke. Always remember to stand in a position where it is easy to lift the cup during the stroke without pulling it away from the tissues. *Always lift or pull, never press or push*, as the latter may inhibit lymph flow. Again, this type of massage lacks sensitivity and can be rather impersonal; therefore the therapist's free hand should follow the cup where possible to maintain some personal contact.

1. Hips and thighs

With the client in a supine position, apply the thin film of oil and choose a small cup (with low pressure) for the inside of the thigh and set the intensity. Stride standing about the level of the client's waist, start at the distal area, i.e. above the patella; let the tissue enter the cup and then slowly draw the cup up the medial (inside) aspect of the thigh to the inguinal nodes. Approximately six strokes can be performed over one pathway before the cup is moved over by half its width to commence the strokes again. As the tissues on the thigh become firmer, the cup should be changed and the intensity increased. Continue across the anterior aspect of the thigh, always finishing the stroke and releasing the vacuum at the inguinal glands (see Fig. 12.1).

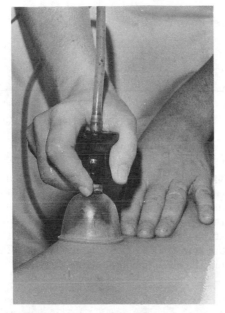

Fig. 12.1 Vacuum suction on the anterior surface of the thigh

For the outer part of the thigh and buttocks, place the client on one side with the knee flexed and the thigh supported. If necessary change the cup and check the intensity. Again start at the distal end and pull the cup forward to the inguinal nodes and using overlapping strokes cover the outside, back of the thigh and buttocks. Where there is considerable adipose tissue present, the strokes should be fast to prevent discomfort for the client and care should be taken coming over the hips to the inguinal nodes to avoid bony areas or separation of the gluteal fold. Figure 12.2 indicates suitable pathways to the inguinal nodes.

Return the client to the supine position and repeat for the other side.

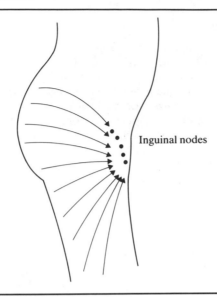

Fig. 12.2 Lateral surface of right upper thigh and buttocks, showing pathways to inguinal nodes

2. Abdomen

With the client lying supine, place a pillow or folded towel under the knees to relax the abdominal muscles. Stand facing the client and, with the correct cup and intensity, start the strokes at the waist area (on the far side) and slowly lift and pull down to the inguinal nodes. Release the vacuum and continue with overlapping strokes across the abdomen (to the waist area on the near side) until the entire area has been completed (see Fig. 12.3). Manual massage to the area could be given to complete the treatment.

3. Midriff

Again with the client lying supine and with a pillow under the knees, stand facing the side of the client. Place a small or medium-size cup on the upper abdominus rectus and let the tissue enter the cup (check the intensity) and following the shape of the rib cage, stroke towards the waist area. The therapist should then alter her stance, change direction of the cup so that it can be pulled upward to the axillary nodes. Care should be taken in the axilla area as the skin can bruise very easily. The number of overlapping strokes that can be made is dependent upon the amount of adipose tissue present and the length of the midriff. The therapist should move to the other side of the couch to repeat the movements (see Fig. 12.3).

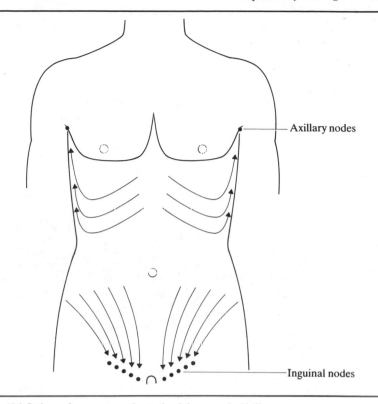

Fig. 12.3 Pathways for vacuum suction to the abdomen and midriff

4. Legs

Vacuum suction can be carried out on the front of the legs with the client lying supine. For the lower leg, a small cup is normally used with a fairly low intensity, starting at the ankle and working round and upward to the popliteal space. Overlapping strokes are taken from either side of the tibia around to the popliteal lymphatic glands. The cup is changed and the intensity increased and vacuum suction is performed on the upper part of the leg (see Fig. 12.4).

The client will lie prone when vacuum suction is given to the back of the legs. Again a small cup and low intensity is used over the lower leg or calf and the strokes are carried to the popliteal lymphatic glands. Often this helps the dispersal of fluid around the ankles and can also help to prevent chilblains and the formation of varicose veins. Fig. 12.4 indicates the pathways for vacuum suction movements for lower and upper legs.

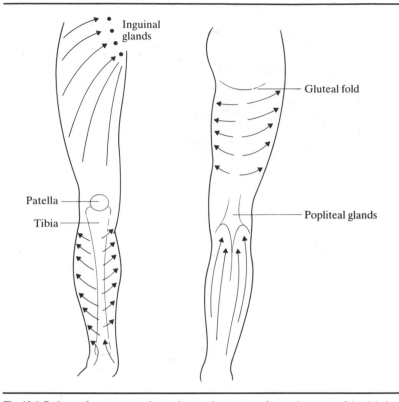

Fig. 12.4 Pathways for vacuum suction to the anterior aspect and posterior aspect of the right leg

5. Arms

The arms are treated in much the same way as the legs. For the forearm vacuum suction is performed, using a very small cup from the wrist to the supratrochlear nodes. For the upper arm, a small to medium cup should be used from above the elbow to the axillary nodes. Figures 12.5 and 12.6 indicate the pathways to the anterior and posterior aspects of the right arm. However, it should be noted that the posterior surface of the upper arm can be included when performing vacuum suction on the back and shoulders.

6. Back and shoulders

With the client lying prone on the couch, ensure that the rest of the body is warm and that there is a pillow under the ankles and, dependent upon the shape and size of the client, a pillow under the abdomen for comfort. If the couch does not have a 'breathing hole' fold a small towel and use as a head

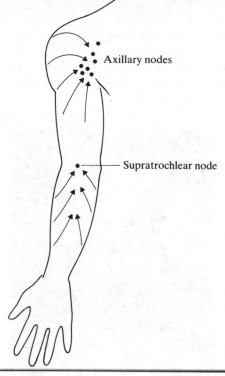

Fig. 12.5 Pathways for vacuum suction to the anterior aspect of the right arm

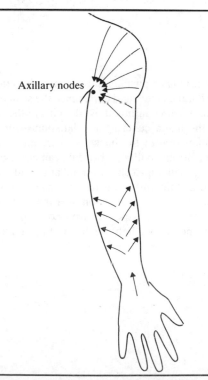

Fig. 12.6 Pathways for vacuum suction to the posterior aspect of the right arm

support. The amount of fat present will determine the cup size, intensity and number of strokes performed, taking into consideration any protruding bones, i.e. scapula, acromion process. To keep the shoulders flat on the couch, it is helpful if the back of the client's hands can rest on the lumbar region (see Fig. 12.7).

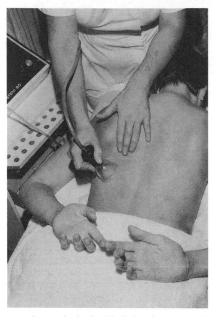

Fig. 12.7 Vacuum suction on the back with the hands resting on the lumbar region

For a pulling, rather than a pushing movement, it is better for the therapist to stand at the head of the couch and commence the strokes from the waist to the axillary nodes and, with continued overlapping of the pathways, from the erector spinae to the axilla covering the latissimus dorsi. This should be repeated for the other side of the back, but care must be exercised not to over-treat the area near the axillae as bruising can easily occur.

For the shoulders the therapist should stand at the side of the couch to pull the stroke from the deltoid and trapezius to the axillary nodes. Figure 12.8 indicates the pathways for vacuum suction over the back and shoulders.

At the end of any treatment, wipe off surplus oil and use a cologne or tonic water over the area and apply a light dusting of talcum power.

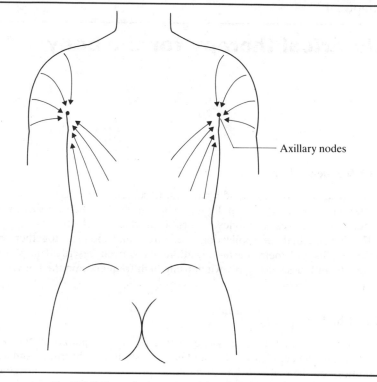

Axillary nodes

Fig. 12.8 Pathways for vacuum suction to the back and shoulders

Maintenance of equipment

The motor/pump is self-lubricating and does not require to be oiled. Always ensure that the edges of the vacuum suction cups remain smooth and free from chips or cracks etc., so that a good vacuum with the skin is formed. The cups should be cleaned with warm soapy water containing an antiseptic. The plastic tubing should be inspected regularly as oily matter can become lodged inside the tubing, usually at each end. To remove this matter, leave the tubing to soak in a hot detergent solution. If the deposits still remain, these may be removed by using an orange stick or by simply cutting off the small amount of tubing involved.

Chapter 13

Electrical therapy for the body

High frequency treatments

High frequency (HF) is a rapidly alternating current in excess of 500 000 Hz (hertz) which oscillates so rapidly that when applied to the skin there is no stimulation of nerves or muscles but heat is produced in the tissues.

The two methods of application, i.e. direct and indirect, together with their benefits and their contra-indications have been described in Vol. 1, Chap. 26, and these also apply when using high frequency on the body.

Direct high frequency

Directly applied high frequency (i.e. with an electrode placed on the skin) has a drying and germicidal effect and is very useful for seborrhoea and acne conditions on the body. Its long-term effect promotes an increase in cellular activity thereby refining the texture of the skin.

Method of treatment

The method of application includes the removal of all jewellery, making the client comfortable, cleansing, toning, drying the area and applying a light dusting of talcum powder. Choose the electrode required, switch on the machine and check that the intensity is at zero. The electrode should be tested on the therapist's arm first and by increasing the intensity the client will be able to observe the light and noise from the electrode and be reassured; the intensity control is then returned to zero.

Place the electrode on the appropriate area, which is usually on the back; increase the intensity until the client can feel a mild, tingling sensation. The pressure and intensity of the current should be consistent with the degree of subcutaneous tissue present and the skin's sensitivity to allow for maximum client comfort. Ensure smooth and even circular movements with a definite pattern, and for the back it is preferable to complete one side, turning down the intensity over the spinous processes before treating the other side. Always avoid any moles or warts that may be present.

Apart from fulguration, which may be applied over certain blemishes with great care being taken to avoid any exacerbation on the area, the electrode must remain in contact with the skin at all times. Application times will vary from 7 to 10 minutes for dry, rough skin using a low intensity, for 10 to 15 minutes for seborrhoeic conditions using a higher intensity.

Turn the intensity control to zero, switch off the machine and remove the electrode from the body. The remains of the talcum powder should be removed with damp cotton wool and the skin patted dry with tissues.

A deeper penetration will be required for aching muscles and joints. This can be obtained by placing two thicknesses of towelling on the skin and, as the electrode moves over the area, the sparks jump a greater distance and penetration is increased (see Fig. 13.1).

Indirect high frequency

Indirect high frequency involves the saturator being held by the client and the hands of the therapist replacing the glass electrode. The method of application includes again the removal of all jewellery and making the client comfortable. The client is requested to hold the saturator with both hands throughout the treatment. The therapist should be careful to avoid touching metal (i.e. arms of chairs). Ensure that the machine is within easy reach and check that the switch is off and that the intensity control is at zero. Talking to the client will enable the therapist not only to dispel nervousness of the treatment but also to judge the client's tolerance level.

The general purpose of indirect frequency massage is either to relieve

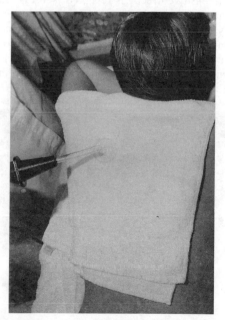

Fig. 13.1 Direct high frequency, deeper penetration using two thicknesses of towelling

tension by giving deep movements or to have a stimulating effect (as lymphatic and venous blood circulation is improved) by giving superficial movements. It can be applied as a general body massage by working around the body, similar to that of manual massage or applied specifically to an area.

Method of treatment

With the client lying supine, take talcum powder or oil to the hands of the therapist and apply to the anterior aspect of the body or to a local area. If oil is used, care will be needed when regulating the intensity control (which may also become greasy) to avoid the fingers slipping on the control. Other preparations may be used, e.g. manufactured ampoules containing specially formulated liquids for specific skin problems.

Place one hand on the client and with the other hand switch on the machine and very slowly turn up the intensity until the client's immediate tolerance level is reached. This hand is then placed on the body for both hands to commence the type of massage required. It is important that one hand remains in contact with the client throughout the treatment as it is essential that no sudden break in the circuit should occur because of the resulting discomfort to both client and therapist. The current intensity can be increased or decreased, providing contact with the client is maintained.

To complete a massage for the body, leave one hand on the client and with the other hand turn the intensity control to zero and remove the saturator from the client. The client turns over and the sequence of using a medium to the posterior surface, placing the saturator in the hands of the client and using the current intensity correctly is repeated (see Fig. 13.2). Should the client experience an unpleasant tingling in the hands when holding the saturator, this is usually caused by perspiration on the skin or possible stiffness in the finger joints and this can be relieved by an application of talcum powder to the palms of the hands.

After the treatment has been completed, the usual care and assistance is given to the client.

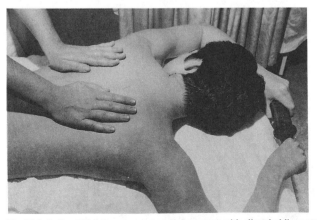

Fig. 13.2 Indirect high frequency on posterior aspect with client holding saturator

Maintenance of the equipment

The maintenance of the equipment is very simple. Leads, plugs and the machine should be checked regularly and the glass electrodes sterilised with surgical spirit before and after use.

Galvanic treatments

Galvanic iontophoresis treatments for the body are becoming popular as a means for treating the soft fat or stubborn fluid fat resembling a 'puffy' distended appearance. The galvanic current, iontophoresis, desincrustation, benefits and some contra-indications have been described in Vol. 1, Chap. 26. Further contra-indications to galvanic iontophoresis for the body would include any condition where there is a lack of sensitivity to heat, defective circulation or hypersensitive areas, i.e. the medial aspect of the thighs or sunburn.

For the body, the electrodes will normally consist of sheets of pliable metal, e.g. tin, and these must be clean and have rounded smooth corners. No metal parts of the electrode should touch the skin as this causes a concentration of current and therefore burning. To prevent this the electrodes must be placed in a foam or viscose envelope which is at least half an inch larger all round the electrode.

By using active substances, e.g. gels, liquids, ampoules etc., under the electrodes an effective result may be achieved. The manufacturers of these substances must state clearly the polarity (− or +) or under which electrode the active substances should be placed.

When using an ampoule, apply the active substance to a square piece of lint and place under the negative pad which is attached to a black lead and inserted into the negative (−) black terminal. Place a similar square of lint, soaked in warm water under the positive pad which is attached to a red lead and inserted into the positive (+) red terminal. The pads are placed on the body and held firmly by elastic straps. The negative electrode, with the active ampoule, being placed on the area to be treated, i.e. where there is cellulite or fatty tissue. The active substance will flow from the negative to the positive electrode, the latter absorbing acid and caustic products of the electrolysis during the treatment. The manufacturer's directions should be followed as to the method of use of the active substance (see Fig. 13.3).

Skin sensitivity may be assessed by way of either ice packs/cubes or hot water or the skin pinch test. A heat treatment or a 5–10 minute massage of the area is beneficial to warm through the tissues, but the medium used must then be removed to provide a clean skin to ensure that the current will not be impeded. During the galvanic treatment the skin's resistance is lowered, therefore the current intensity may need reducing to prevent any discomfort. Due to the localised stimulation of the circulation, it is normal for a slight reddening of the area to occur but if this is excessive the treatment must be terminated.

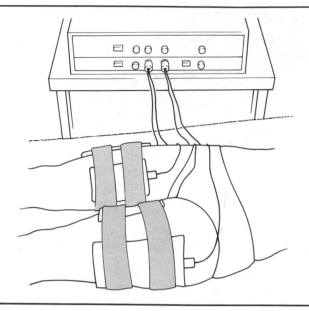

Fig. 13.3 Galvanic treatment showing placement of electrodes

Method of treatment

Ensure the client is comfortable and all jewellery removed. Check the machine: the indicator must be in the 'off' position, the intensity control at zero. The machine is then switched on and the intensity slowly increased from zero until a prickling sensation is felt, followed by a general feeling of warmth from the positive electrode. The therapist should converse with the client to ensure a comfortable treatment.

If for any reason the circuit is broken between an electrode and the body, e.g. if the voltage supply is cut off, there will be an unpleasant electric shock which could also cause sudden muscle contraction. Obviously the current should be immediately switched off but fortunately this is very rare as modern machines have safety factors built in. In most cases, where the treatment feels uncomfortable, all that is required is for the intensity control to be returned to zero and brought up again slowly.

Galvanic current itself will not cause a burn but if there is a concentration of alkali or acid formed, a chemical burn may occur. This is recognised by the area appearing grey in colour or a series of grey spots. Should this happen wash the affected area with plenty of cold water and cover with a dry dressing. Never leave the client, and watch the intensity of the current; as already explained, this may increase when the skin's resistance is lowered as the active substances penetrate through to the underlying tissues.

The first treatment should be for 10 minutes and increased to 25–30 minutes for subsequent treatments. At the end of the treatment the intensity control is reduced slowly to zero, the machine is turned off and straps, leads and pads are removed from the client. Wash and dry the area and massage the skin to remove any toxins and waste. Again check the manufacturer's instructions as there may be a reason to follow with gels or creams to complete the treatment.

Finally, ensure that the usual care and assistance is given to the client before leaving the salon.

The lint and foam/sponge envelopes must be washed thoroughly and dried after use.

Faradic treatments

The faradic current is an interrupted direct current producing groups of short pulses of current separated by intervals when no current flows. As explained in Vol. 1 Chap. 26, all nervous and muscular activity is caused by minute electrical currents originating in the brain passing along nerves causing muscles to contract, i.e. motor nerves of the cerebrospinal system. A surged faradic-type current or EMS (electronic muscle stimulation) will produce a similar effect; contracting muscles without the participation of the client and resembling natural muscular exercise.

The faradic current can be applied to the body in two ways: by using an active button electrode on the motor point of one muscle at a time or by using semi-conductor pads on a group of muscles. The former (explained in Vol. 1, Chap. 26) is very time-consuming and is rarely used in a clinic situation for body treatments. Faradic machines vary in size with corresponding outlets. The smaller units have 4 outlets with 8 pads and are ideal for a home visiting practice or for home use, but clinic models usually have 6–8 outlets providing 12–16 pads.

The only slight disadvantage with the smaller units is the fact that they are not as powerful as their salon counterparts. It is admitted by some manufacturers that the current intensity will not be strong enough to contract all the muscles properly, therefore it is important to have a demonstration and try out the unit before purchase.

Designs vary with each manufacturer and, although the principle remains the same, some are slightly more sophisticated than others by incorporating a wider range of different controls to alter the form of the programme. At the present time, machines are being developed to include the most up-to-date research on muscle exercise with advanced computerised systems enabling the therapist to choose from the six programmes available or devising and storing a programme for a specific purpose.

It is probably helpful to describe one clinic unit which is currently in general use. It has 9 slide controls, 8 of which connect with 8 leads and 8 pairs of body pads. Each of the 8 leads plug into a recessed socket. The 9th slide control, namely the 'Master Output %', increases the pulse width equally across all the 8 pairs of pads when it is advanced and there is a general feeling of increased intensity of muscle contraction.

A 'safe start' device is built in to ensure that all the slide controls are in an 'off' position before commencement of the treatment. A red 'reset' light glows if any of the slide controls are left on but when these are returned to the 'off' position this light will go out and a green 'ready' light will start flashing on and off to signify that the machine is ready for further use. The built-in digital timer simply assists the therapist to control the client's treatment time.

TENS (Transcutaneous Electric Nerve Stimulation) is another feature built into the unit which is said to 'anaesthetise' the area being treated against discomfort. The client will feel the TENS sensation as a very slight tingling on the skin throughout the treatment. (On the new machines a sub-pulse is added to smooth out the contraction at low frequencies.)

There is also a pad-movement facility which means that the therapist can move the pads on the body during the treatment without any discomfort to the client. Each pair of pads is isolated from all other pairs to obviate any inter-reaction between them.

This particular machine has a *mono-phasic wave form* which, if used correctly, is more comfortable than the by-phasic form. With the mono-phasic form the impulse flows in one direction only from negative to positive and therefore one pad of the pair is $(-)$ and the other $(+)$. The positive pad is

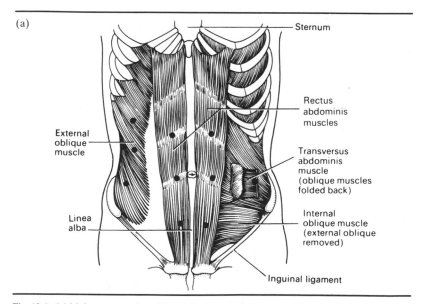

(a)

Sternum

Rectus abdominis muscles

External oblique muscle

Transversus abdominis muscle (oblique muscles folded back)

Internal oblique muscle (external oblique removed)

Linea alba

Inguinal ligament

Fig. 13.4 (a) Major motor points of the abdomen

(b)

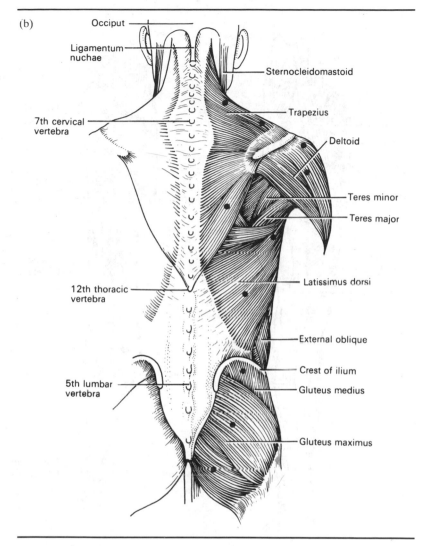

Fig. 13.4 (b) Major motor points of the back

always placed on the most sensitive area and the therapist can identify this pad as it is at the end of the 'ridged' side of the lead. The negative pad is placed on a less sensitive area. Whereas the bi-phasic form, having a resistor inside the unit, constantly changes the flow of current so that both pads become alternately positive and negative.

There is a choice of frequencies from 100 through to 80 and to 60. It is

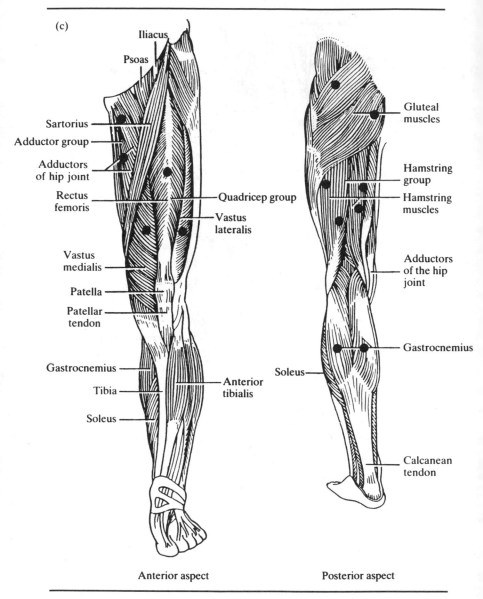

(c)

Iliacus

Psoas

Sartorius

Adductor group

Adductors
of hip joint

Rectus
femoris

Vastus
medialis

Patella

Patellar
tendon

Gastrocnemius

Tibia

Soleus

Quadricep group

Vastus
lateralis

Anterior
tibialis

Gluteal
muscles

Hamstring
group

Hamstring
muscles

Adductors
of the hip
joint

Gastrocnemius

Soleus

Calcanean
tendon

Anterior aspect

Posterior aspect

Fig. 13.4 (c) Major motor points of the legs

always advisable to start with 100, which gives a light massaging effect with superficial contraction, before proceeding to 80 for an intermediate contraction and then to 60 for deep muscle contraction. When working through the frequencies there is always a very slight increase or decrease felt in the intensity of the muscle contraction; therefore the therapist should reduce or increase either the intensity slide controls or the 'Master Output %' for client comfort.

Contraction and relaxation times depend entirely on the type of muscle being treated; therefore the therapist should examine the condition of the muscles before deciding on the contraction time. If the relaxation time is too short the muscle will tire and there will be a build-up of lactic acid which may lead to cramp.

In order to provide a good comfortable treatment an in-depth knowledge of the anatomy of the muscles is required and also a knowledge of the motor points is desirable (see Fig. 13.4 (a) to (c)). The positioning of the pads is very important. They should be placed either over the motor point (i.e. the point at which the motor nerve actually supplies and enters the muscle) or the more general use where a pair of pads are placed near to the origin and insertion of the muscle group to receive a maximum concentration of current through them. Manufacturers will often supply padding lay-outs but the therapist should be able to select those which are the most suitable for the client following muscle groups which require exercise.

The benefits and effects of EMS

For the body, the benefits (other than those for the face) are:

- a reduction of inches where figure shaping is required, i.e. toning muscles on thighs or buttocks when these are out of proportion to the rest of the figure;
- improving the waistline when this has become thickened;
- toning the pectoral muscles, particularly after breast feeding;
- to re-educate poor muscle tone, which is usually due to lack or incorrect use of the muscles;
- and to maintain a firm figure.

It should be remembered that muscles are a bundle of elastic fibres which retain their elasticity when used, but lack of use makes them flabby and longer.

The following are some of the effects of EMS:

- to increase metabolism with a consequent demand for oxygen and food-stuffs by the muscle being exercised and an increased output of waste products including metabolites;
- the metabolites cause dilation of capillaries and arterioles and so there is a considerable increase in blood supply to the muscle;

- by contracting and relaxing, the muscles exert a pumping action on the surrounding veins and lymphatic vessels;
- adhesions that have formed are stretched and loosened by this action;
- it can also be used for injured or weak muscles providing there is no rupture present.

Contra-indications to EMS

- Any client wearing a pace-maker (due to the possibility of interference); a history of thrombosis or phlebitis;
  defective circulation from systemic causes;
  spastic or muscular disorders, i.e. multiple sclerosis, (unless medical approval has been given);
  epilepsy;
  any part of the body which is inflamed through disease or injury unless medical approval is given;
  not over varicose veins;
  hernia;
  not after operations or recent scar tissue;
  not over the abdomen during the first two days of menstruation;
  pregnancy and not immediately after pregnancy – leave for six months before starting treatment;
  renal conditions;
- if, for medical reasons, the client has been advised against normal exercise, medical approval should be sought.

Preparation

Ensure that the machine is on a stable trolley or surface and plug into a socket (some machines may be battery-operated and the latter will not apply).

For ease of pad identification, leads of the same colour should be plugged into adjacent sockets, thereby the pads attached to matching colour leads can be placed on the opposite side of the body.

The skin of the area to be treated should be clean, i.e. free from oils or creams, and the tissues warmed through by a heat treatment, e.g. sauna, steam cabinet, infra-red lamp or sunbed.

A bowl of warm saline solution should be close to hand but not put on top of the machine.

- Place the elastic body and/or limb straps on the couch with the hooking ends of the velcro uppermost.

As with most slimming treatments, the client's medical history should be checked for contra-indications. If a course of treatment is indicated, measurements should be taken to assess loss of inches. Always advise the

Faradic treatments - suggested area to be measured												
CLIENT'S NAME					OPERATOR'S NAME							
DATE												
WEIGHT												
CHEST (at armpit)												
UPPER ARM (middle) R												
L												
DIAPHRAGM												
WAIST												
UPPER HIP (3" below waist)												
LOWER HIP (top of hair line)												
BUTTOCKS (widest point)												
UPPER THIGH R												
(as high as possible) L												
MIDDLE THIGH R												
(7" above knee) L												
LOWER THIGH R												
(1" above knee) L												

Fig. 13.5 Areas to be measured.

client that there will not be a weight reduction unless combined with dietary control and physical exercise. Figure 13.5 shows the areas to be measured.

Method of treatment

● The client should lie on top of the straps in a comfortable semi-reclining position, with a pillow under the knees, if the anterior/medial/lateral aspects of the body or limbs are to be treated; or with pillows for the abdomen, forehead and under the ankles if the posterior aspect is to be treated. This will allow maximum muscle relaxation (see Figs 13.6 and 13.7).

● The elastic straps are fastened around the area to be treated. The machine is then switched on with all controls in an 'off' position.

● Take the first pair of pads and to moisten them, either immerse them in the bowl of warm saline solution or use a wet sponge or cotton wool; be careful not to allow the solution to drip over the client as it cools very quickly and will feel very cold to the skin.

● Having decided the padding lay-out, place the pads in pairs over the muscle motor points (or insertion and origin of muscles) with the black granular side of the pads held firmly against the skin by the straps.

● When all the pads are in place ensure that these are correctly positioned and that the whole surface of the pad is in contact with the skin.

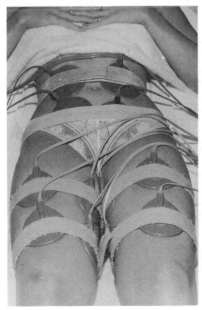

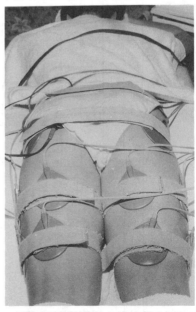

Fig. 13.6 Faradic padding for the abdomen, adductors and quadricep muscles

Fig. 13.7 Faradic padding for gluteals and hamstring muscles

● Check the condition of the muscles and choose the appropriate frequency.

● Advance very slowly the slide control for each pair of pads and observe the action of the muscles being treated. Sometimes a contraction of any sort may not be seen initially; therefore it is important to converse with the client for any reaction. When all the pads being used are working they should be in unison, but as all muscles have varying tone it may be necessary to increase/decrease the intensity of impulse by using one or more slide controls to achieve a balanced degree of exercise.

● Observe the muscle contractions achieved as it may be necessary either to alter the contraction and relaxation times, or slightly adjust the position of either pad.

● If there is an unpleasant tingling sensation, check that the pads and the area are clean, the conducting surfaces of the pads are wet and that all the pads are firmly held against the skin.

● Work through the various frequencies, ensuring each time the comfort of the client and finish the treatment with a frequency of 100.

● On completion of the treatment, which should last about 30–45 minutes, the impulses will stop and the 'reset' light will glow red. All the slide controls should be moved to the 'off' position and then the green light will appear. The machine should be unplugged from the wall (if necessary) should the machine not be required again. Straps are removed from the client and the pads put to one side. Apply an astringent or toner to the area treated, pat dry and finally assist the client from the couch.

Should an occasion arise where the client shows a sensitivity to rubber, this can be overcome by the use of a circle of lint, slightly larger than the pad, thoroughly wetted with water and placed between the skin and the rubber pad.

It is not possible to reshape a client who is considerably overweight and it is better to advise alternative treatments and suggest a good reducing diet and isometric exercises.

Maintenance of equipment

Always wash the pads after each treatment with mild soapy water, never use detergent or spirit. With constant use the pads will deteriorate and will need replacing, i.e. if bald patches appear on the granular surface of the pad or a pad has a wavy edge. Ensure that the leads remain untangled at all times as bent leads cause the plastic covering to crack and these will then need to be replaced. It is wise to obtain spares or replacements from the manufacturer of the machine.

Faradic and galvanic current

There are also machines available carrying these two currents where the combination of faradic stimulation and iontophoresis can aid the breakdown of fat. It is important that the therapist is trained by the manufacturer of these machines and also in the use of their accompanying products.

Interferential current

Another method of stimulating muscle fibres and increasing circulation is the use of the *interferential current*. This current consists of two low-frequency currents which are crossed and literally interfere with each other. The point at which they cross in the body produces the above physical effects in the tissues. In the main it is used for sport injuries, torn ligaments etc., and generally used by specialists in this field such as physiotherapists. As yet, it does not appear to have a wide use in the beauty salon.

Chapter 14

Paraffin wax and parafango wax therapy

Paraffin wax

Paraffin wax baths have been described in Vol. 1, Chap. 30, together with the application to the hand or foot. Paraffin wax as a full body bath provides a relaxing, deep penetrating heat.

The effects of paraffin wax

Apart from the above, paraffin wax:

- has the therapeutic effect of promoting sweating which helps to draw excess fluids and toxins from the body;
- holds its heat, which is readily acceptable to the body, to help soothe tension and ease aches and pains;
- is an effective treatment for clients with arthritic or rheumatic conditions;
  assists in the healing of minor injuries, i.e. sprains or strains, bursitis and contusions;
- penetrates the tissues to relieve stiffness in joints;
- relaxes muscles.

Contra-indications to paraffin wax

Skin diseases, including athletes foot;
cuts and abrasions;
pustular areas;
warts or moles of a suspicious nature;
varicose veins or varicose ulcers;
hypersensitive skin, sunburn or windburn;
diabetes.

As there is a build-up of warmth in the body, similar to the steam cabinet and sauna, the contra-indications for these should also be taken into account.

Preparation for a full body bath

Ensure that the room is warm. The couch or plinth should be covered with two blankets and a towel which is protected by disposable paper. On top of these place about three sheets of polythene and another sheet should be put around the couch to protect the floor covering. An infra-red lamp or a heated electric blanket/s should be to hand and the paraffin wax melted to 49°C (120°F). A large brush is also required for the application. Another method still being used is to whisk the melted wax and apply with the hands all over the body. When the client arrives and starts to undress, turn on the infra-red lamp or electric blankets to warm the wrappings on the couch to ensure maximum heat at the start of the treatment.

Method of use

1. Give the client a shower cap to put on. The therapist should wear some protective clothing, e.g. a plastic apron.
2. Settle the client comfortably on the polythene sheeting on one side of the body with the posterior aspect facing the therapist.
3. Place a strip of tissue between the client's legs to protect the pubic area and gluteal fold. If the client is very hairy, especially on the chest or back, place a large paper tissue over the area before applying the wax as it is very difficult to remove wax from the hairs without discomfort.
4. The temperature of the wax should be tested on the inside of the wrist of the therapist before application and the procedure should be explained to the client.
5. Apply the wax from the soles of the feet, working up the back of the legs. The wax will set immediately but use several coats, i.e. 4–5 applications to form a good layer. Continue painting in wide strips from the cervical area down the back and any wax drips that trickle down will be incorpor-

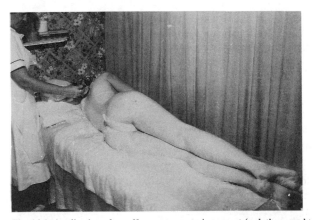

Fig. 14.1 Application of paraffin wax to posterior aspect (polythene and towels removed)

ated in the application of the next strip. Again form a good layer (see Fig. 14.1).

6. When this has been completed the client turns supine and the chest and abdomen are covered with a towel for warmth. Apply the wax from the toes to the groin, taking care to ensure that there are no gaps in the coating. The thighs must have a good covering as this is the area where fluid is most likely to collect. The therapist should work quickly to make certain that the wax remains as hot as possible.

7. Wrapping the feet and legs follows by folding the polythene sheeting over the area and covering it with a towel and blanket. Position the lamp (or electric blanket) to heat the treated area.

8. Lift the client's arm and, with palm uppermost, cover well with wax to the shoulder and then apply the wax to the sides and back of the arm. Fold in the polythene and blanket and repeat the procedure for the other arm. Regularly check the temperature of the wax and that the client is comfortable.

9. Remove the towel from the abdomen and check that the pubic area is still protected by paper tissues. Generously apply the wax to the hips, waist and abdomen. Remove the towel from the chest and continue waxing from this area to the clavicle, again ensuring that there are no gaps in the coating, except over the area of the heart.

10. Complete the wrapping process; tuck the blanket in firmly, especially around the neck area, to prevent the heat escaping. Place cool eyepads over the client's eyes and re-position the lamp (or electric blanket/s) on the body. Always check at regular intervals to ensure that the client is comfortable and refreshen eyepads. Do not leave the area as some clients may find this treatment claustrophobic.

11. After 30 minutes the client should be sweating freely and the wrappings may be removed. Leave the lamp (or an electric blanket) in position to keep the client warm and unwrap the feet and legs. Run a thumb from the toes to the hips (see Fig. 14.2) to split the wax coating, which will be

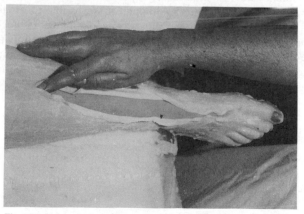

Fig. 14.2 Removal of paraffin wax (starting at the toes)

soft and malleable, and peel it off each side of the leg. Continue in this way for the arms and anterior aspect of the body. The client should then sit up for the therapist to remove the wax from the back and ensure that all traces of wax have been removed from the body. Wrap the client in towels and advise a warm shower.

12. Often there are pools of water on the polythene sheeting which should be mopped up before placing the sheeting in the waste bin, together with all the used paraffin wax. The latter must not be melted to use again as it will contain sweat and body toxins. Place all towels in the laundry basket and remove the polythene sheeting from the floor.

The whole process will take about an hour, i.e. allow 15 minutes for the application of the wax, 30 minutes for the treatment and the balance to remove the wax and clear the area.

Maintenance of equipment

There is very little maintenance for the paraffin wax bath itself but the thermostat should be checked at regular intervals. Any residue of wax left in the bath, however clean, should be removed periodically and the bath washed out, just in case any impurities are transferred from the brush to the existing wax. The brush itself should be cleaned after use.

Parafango wax

The wax is a potent curative mud, almost black in colour and comes from the ash of volcanic mountains or from certain thermal lakes and seas. It can contain among other things: silica, alumina, lime, manganese sulphur, iron oxides, titanium oxide, soda, potash, copper salts, organic matter and traces of iodine, in variable quantities. Although it is possible to obtain 'fango' powder it is usually mixed with paraffin wax as 'parafango' in blocks of 1 or 2 kg (approximately 2 or 4 lb). In block form it will retain all its properties and is re-usable for at least 25 treatments and, at the temperatures recommended, it is self-sterilising. The wax can be melted and used for certain areas or used as a full body treatment.

The effects of parafango wax

- Its heat retaining properties mean that it produces dilation of the blood vessels and erythema of the tissues;
- increased blood circulation;
- sweating can be induced;
- intra cellular fluid dissipated;

- pain in joints and muscles relieved;
  helps the breaking down of cellulite and fatty tissue.

Contra-indications to parafango wax

Heart and circulatory defects;
active pulmonary tuberculosis;
thrombosis;
diabetes;
pregnancy;
and similar contra-indications to the use of paraffin wax.

Preparation

The fango blocks are preheated in a thermostatically controlled wax bath (i.e. the same type as used for paraffin wax) or melted in special ovens on trays with plastic sheeting underlays. For the first treatment the temperature is kept at 46–57°C or 114–134°F and for subsequent treatments the temperature can be raised slightly to 60°C or 140°F. Assuming that a wax bath is used, when the fango has melted to a semi-liquid, it can be taken out of the bath with a large spatula and spread out on a sheet of plastic, levelling it out to a thickness of about half an inch and the desired width. After a few minutes the fango will go from a shiny to a dull appearance and, when tested with the fingers, there will be indentations (see Fig. 14.3). It is then ready to place on the client but a test should be made on the therapist's wrist first.

Method of use

For use on certain areas only – ensure the client is wrapped up in towels with only the area to be treated exposed. For example, for the knee, take the

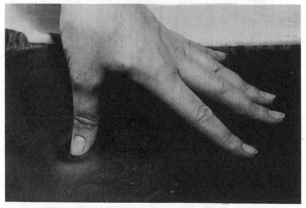

Fig. 14.3 Parafango wax laid out on a sheet of plastic

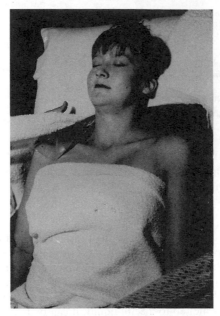

Fig. 14.4 Application of parafango on the back

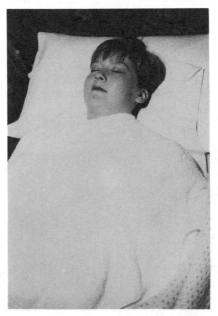

Fig. 14.5 Method of wrapping towels following use of parafango wax

prepared wax and wrap the whole leg from the foot; for the hips (using paper tissues in the gluteal fold and over the pubic area), lay the client on the wax and bring the wax right round to meet at the pubic area; for the thighs use two pieces of prepared wax and wrap around each thigh; for the shoulders, ensure that the wax covers the scapula and well over the acromion processes and for the back (see Fig. 14.4).

With these examples the therapist should be able to arrange the placement of the wax in any area required. One can always introduce an essential oil on gauze next to the skin before applying the wax (for instance a few drops of fennel, rosemary or juniper in an almond base for cellulite), as the heat would aid the penetration of the oil. The client should then be firmly wrapped in towels (see Fig. 14.5) and blankets and left for approximately 35 minutes. At the end of the treatment time, when the wrapping is undone the therapist will find that the parafango wax has hardened and can be lifted off in one piece.

For a full body treatment (without total immersion in a bath) lie the client on plastic sheeting prone, apply from foot to thigh and then on the back and follow as for a full body paraffin wax treatment.

Do not leave the client; always ensure that he/she is comfortable, and if necessary unwrap an arm or the chest to give a sense of freedom. The use of a thermal blanket or lamp is not required as parafango wax will retain a constant temperature during the treatment.

Maintenance of equipment

There is virtually no maintenance required, only the thermostat needs checking at regular intervals. The wax itself is re-usable, but it is suggested that it is thrown away after 25 treatments.

Chapter 15

Aromatherapy and reflexology

Aromatherapy is a treatment that combines specialised massage techniques using essential (aromatic) oils on the nerve centres of the body and head.

The origins of aromatherapy date back some 4000 years and today's practical application of the essential oils of plants and flowers help to maintain or restore natural harmony in the human body. To understand this further the following explains the natural life force of the body and of the plants used for aromatherapy to achieve a complete balance.

Life force

It is important to appreciate that every living thing has a life force (or energy) which is a balance between positive and negative (or passive and active). One cannot touch, smell or analyse it and in Western countries we are inclined to think of this life force in terms of *energy* continually bringing about a state of health and harmony. In India it is called *Prana* and in China, *Ch'i*, but whatever it is called it is the essence of every living thing.

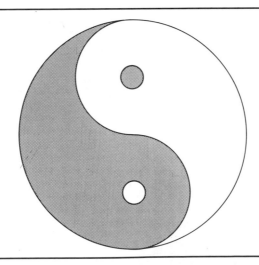

Fig. 15.1 Shape symbol of Yin and Yang

There are two Oriental words, Yin and Yang, which are better suited to describe the balance of life force as they are not so definitive as negative and positive. Nothing is totally Yin or totally Yang although they are traditionally opposite. They always have a complete balance; for example, a seed needs earth (Yang) and water (Yin) to grow. Fig. 15.1. shows the 'S' shape representing the two qualities balancing within each other.

The life force or personality of a plant varies during each day or season and this affects the essential oil cells which are distributed throughout the flowers or leaves or stems or roots in minute odiferous droplets. It is this life force of the plant which we introduce into the body by aromatherapy. Most essential oils are Yang (see Table 15.1.) but they will always contain certain Yin properties.

Table 15.1   Yin and Yang oils

Yang oils	*Yin oils*
Basil	Camomile
Benzoin	Camphor
Bergamot	Cypress
Black pepper	Eucalyptus
Cardamon	Geranium
Cedarwood	Rose
Clary sage	Ylang-ylang
Fennel	
Frankincense	
Hyssop	
Jasmine	
Juniper	
Lavender	
Lemon	
Marjoram	
Melissa	
Myrrh	
Neroli	
Patchouli	
Pennyroyal	
Peppermint	
Rosemary	
Sandalwood	

Properties and effects of essential oils

1. Aromatherapy differs from herbalism in as much as that it only uses a special part of the plant or herb whereas herbalism uses the whole. This special part is the essence of the plant or herb and is called the 'essential' oil. Essential oils are extracted from a particular part of the plant, for example, from:

   bark   –   cinnamon, cascarilla
   flowers   –   lavender, orange-blossom, rose, ylang-ylang
   fruit   –   citron, juniper, nutmeg, orange
   herbs   –   hyssop, marjoram, melissa, patchouli

leaves – bay, eucalytus, thyme

wood – cedarwood, pine, rosewood, sandalwood.

2. Although the chemistry of the oils is complex, they usually contain alcohols, esters, ketones, aldehydes and terpenes.

3. Most oils are said to have antiseptic, healing and curative properties and only the smallest amount is necessary to correct the balance of the body and tissue.

4. Essential oils are volatile and fall into three categories according to their evaporation rate. Using a simple table 1–100:

   Top notes (1–14) are the lightest and evaporate the fastest (e.g. eucalyptus). They are usually the most stimulating and uplifting to mind and body.

   Middle notes (15–60) are moderately volatile and the aroma lasts for approximately 2–3 days (e.g. geranium). These primarily affect the digestive functions of the body and metabolism. It is important to include one middle note in all compositions to ensure a link between fast and slow elements, i.e. between air and earth.

   Base notes (61–100) are slower to evaporate, i.e. a lower volatility (e.g. sandalwood) and the aroma can last for at least a week. These can also be used as fixatives to hold back the scent of other aromatic oils. They are the most sedative and relaxing. Table 15.2 gives an approximate volatility rate for a number of essential oils.

5. Essential oils are used in carrier oils for massage and added to water for baths, inhalation and compresses. Alcohol, due to its quick evaporation has the property of making the oil too fluid

6. The power of penetration of essential oils through the pores of the skin is such that it is passed through the epidermis and dermis into the intracellular fluids. It then becomes absorbed through the capillary and lymphatic network into the general circulation. Absorption time varies between 25 and 70 minutes.

7. Certain oils are cytophylactic (i.e. promote the growth of new cells).

8. Some oils have draining and diuretic properties and certain oils can also be used as a regulator of waste products.

   Elimination of the oils can take place in a number of ways, through the urine (if they are soluble in water) or excreted into the intestinal tract via the bile and so eliminated in the faeces, as well as through the lungs, saliva, tears, sweat and even milk.

9. Oils can be used for either stimulation or relaxation.

10. Olfaction plays an important role in aromatherapy; therefore the intensity of odours is important when mixing oils. One oil may over-power all others when its intensity is high (e.g. camomile) and the amount of each oil used should be carefully considered. Table 15.2 gives an approximate odour intensity for some of the oils.

11. Effects of essential oils on the skin are:
    - *antiseptic* (bergamot, eucalyptus, juniper);
    - *cooling effect* by constricting the capillaries and reducing high colour (camomile, cypress, peppermint);

- *stimulating the circulation*, so nourishing and feeding the skin (benzoin, camphor, geranium, juniper, rosemary);
- *relaxing effect* (jasmine, marjoram, neroli, rose, sandalwood).

Floral oils have their main effect on the olfactory nerve endings. For easy reference some essential oils, their use for massage and odour intensity are detailed in Table 15.2.

Extraction, use of oils and storage

Methods to extract essential oils.

Distillation   which involves boiling water or steam being passed through the flowers or plants and the vapours condensed through a still.

Solvent   extraction, where plants are left in a liquid solvent to dissolve the essential oil. Subsequently this is evaporated at a low temperature and finally passed through alcohol. This method is expensive but is used where precious oils can be destroyed by heat.

Enfleurage and maceration   where the fruits and skins of fruits are pressed between sheets of glass into hot and cold fats – though these are methods rarely used now.

This is a very limited outline of the extraction of essential oils as most therapists purchase their oils already bottled by reputable suppliers.

The quality of the oil depends on the soil, climate and method of cultivation and time and method of harvesting. This varies a great deal in different parts of the world.

Use of oils

Essential oils can be used in many ways:

- inhalation and vaporisation in a facial steamer;
- bathing, where drops of oils are added to bath water;
- compresses, packs and masks;
- external absorption by massage and electrical means (i.e. ionisation);
- internally, as herbal teas or infusions.

Essential oils should not be used 'neat' on the skin. There are one or two that can 'burn' the skin (i e the citrus group) or cause irritation or allergy. For a list of proscribed oils, see Table 15.3. Only small quantities of essential oils are used. Two or three oils may be blended into a carrier oil, e.g. basic vegetable oils such as sweet almond, avocado, grapeseed, hazelnut or wheatgerm.

Table 15.2 Some essential oils which can be used for aromatherapy massage

Problem	Top notes	Odour intensity	Middle notes	Odour intensity	Base notes	Odour intensity
Allergies	eucalyptus for respiratory tract	8	camomile	9		
			melissa	4		
Alopecia			lavender	4		
			rosemary	6		
Anaemia	lemon	7	camomile	9		
Arteriosclerosis			juniper	5		
			rosemary	6		
Asthma	eucalyptus	8	cypress	4	benzoin	4
			hyssop	6		
			lavender	4		
			marjoram	5		
			melissa	4		
			peppermint	7		
			rosemary	6		
Bronchitis	basil	7	cardamon	9	benzoin	4
	bergamot	4	hyssop	6	cedarwood	4
	eucalyptus	8	rosemary	6	frankincense	7
			lavender	5		
			peppermint	7	sandalwood	5
Bruises			camphor	5		
			hyssop	6		
Burns	eucalyptus	8	camomile	9		
			camphor	5		
			lavender	4		
			geranium	6		
			rosemary	6		

Ailment	Oil	No.	Oils	No.	Oils	No.
Catarrh	eucalyptus	8	hyssop	6	cedarwood	4
			lavender	4	frankincense	7
					myrrh	7
					sandalwood	5
Cellulitis			juniper	5		
			lavender	4		
			rosemary	6		
Cellulite			fennel	6		
			juniper	5		
			rosemary	6		
Chilblains	lemon	7	cypress	4		
			lavender	4		
Circulation (general)			geranium	6		
Cirrhosis			fennel	6	rose	7
Colds	basil	7	black pepper	7		
	eucalyptus	8	camphor	5		
			marjoram	5		
			melissa	4		
			peppermint	7		
			rosemary	6		
Colitis	bergamot	4	black pepper	7	neroli	5
			camomile	9	ylang-ylang	6
			lavender	4		
			rosemary	6		
Conjunctivitis (use as eye compress)			camomile	9	rose	7
			lavender	4		
Constipation			black pepper	7	rose	7
			camphor	5		
			fennel	6		
			hyssop	6		
			marjoram	5		

cont'd

Problem	Top notes	Odour intensity	Middle notes	Odour intensity	Base notes	Odour intensity
Coughs	eucalyptus	8	black pepper	7	benzoin	4
			cardamon	9	jasmine	7
			cypress	4	myrrh	7
			frankincense	7		
			hyssop	6	sandalwood	5
			juniper	5		
			peppermint	5		
Cystitis	bergamot	4	juniper	5	cedarwood	4
	eucalyptus	8	lavender	4	sandalwood	5
Depression	basil	7	camomile	9	jasmine	7
	bergamot	4	camphor	5	neroli	5
	clary-sage	5	geranium	6	patchouli	5
			lavender	4	rose	7
			melissa	4	sandalwood	5
					ylang-ylang	6
Diabetes	eucalyptus	8	geranium	6		
	lemon	7	juniper	5		
			rosemary	6		
Diarrhoea	eucalyptus	8	black pepper	7	myrrh	7
			camomile	9	neroli	5
			cypress	4	sandalwood	5
			geranium	6	nutmeg	6
			lavender	4		
			peppermint	7		
			rosemary	6		
Epilepsy	basil	7	lavender	4		
			rosemary	6		

Condition						
Fainting	basil	7	black pepper	7	myrrh	7
	bergamot	4	camomile	9		
	sage	5	lavender	4		
			melissa	4		
			peppermint	7		
			rosemary	6		
Flatulence	bergamot	4	black pepper	7		
	clary sage	5	camomile	9		
			camphor	5		
			cardamon	9		
			fennel	6		
			hyssop	6		
			juniper	5		
			lavender	4		
			marjoram	5		
			peppermint	7		
			rosemary	6		
Fluid retention	eucalyptus	8	fennel	6	benzoin	4
	sage	5	geranium	6	patchouli	5
			lavender	4		
			rosemary	6		
Gall stones	bergamot	4	camphor	5	ylang-ylang	6
	eucalyptus	8	lavender	4		
			peppermint	7		
			rosemary	6		
Gout	basil	7	camomile	9	benzoin	4
			camphor	5		
			juniper	5		
Halitosis	bergamot	4	cardamon	9	myrrh	7
			lavender	4		
			peppermint	7		

cont'd

Problem	Top notes	Odour intensity	Middle notes	Odour intensity	Base notes	Odour intensity
Headaches	lemon	7	camomile	9		
			cardamon	9	rose	7
			lavender	4		
			marjoram	5		
			peppermint	7		
			rosemary	6		
Heartburn			black pepper	7		
			cardamon	9		
Haemorrhoids (piles)			cypress	4		
			juniper	5		
Hepatitis			rosemary	6		
Hyperglycaemia			rosemary	6		
Hypertension	clary-sage	5	hyssop	6	ylang-ylang	6
			lavender	4		
			marjoram	5		
			melissa	4		
Hypotension	sage	5	camphor	5		
	thyme	6	hyssop	6		
			rosemary	6		
Hysteria	basil	7	camomile	9	neroli	5
	clary sage	5	camphor	5		
			hyssop	6		
			lavender	4		
			marjoram	5		
			peppermint	7		
			rosemary	6		

Ailment			
Indigestion	basil 7 bergamot 4 clary sage 5 eucalyptus 8	black pepper 7 camomile 9 cardamon 9 fennel 6 hyssop 6 juniper 5 lavender 4 melissa 4 peppermint 7 rosemary 6	frankincense 7 myrrh 7 origanum 5
Influenza	eucalyptus 8	blackpepper 7 hyssop 6 lavender 4 peppermint 7 rosemary 6 cypress 4	
Insomnia	basil 7	camphor 5 camomile 9 lavender 4 marjoram 5	neroli 5 rose 7 sandalwood 5 ylang-ylang 6
Jaundice		geranium 6 rosemary 6	
Kidney (general problems)	clary sage 5 eucalyptus	juniper 5	cedarwood 4 sandalwood 5
Laryngitis	lavender 4	lavender 4	benzoin 4 frankincense 7 sandalwood 5
Loss of voice		cypress 4 lavender 4	

cont'd

Problem	Top notes	Odour intensity	Middle notes	Odour intensity	Base notes	Odour intensity
Menopause			camomile	9		
			cypress	4		
			fennel	6		
Menstruation						
amenorrhoea	clary	5	camomile	9	myrrh	7
			fennel	6		
			hyssop	6		
			juniper	5		
dysmenorrhoea	clary	5	camomile	9	jasmine	7
			cypress	4		
			juniper	5		
			marjoram	5		
			melissa	4		
			peppermint	7		
			rosemary	6		
irregular	clary	5	melissa	4	rose	7
Mental fatigue	basil	7	cardamon	9		
			peppermint	7		
			rosemary	6		
Migraine	basil	7	camomile	9		
	eucalyptus	8	lavender	4		
			marjoram	5		
			melissa	4		
			peppermint	7		
			rosemary	6		
Nausea	basil	7	black pepper	7		
			cardoman	9		
			fennel	6		
			lavender	4		
			melissa	4		

Condition	Oil	No.	Oil	No.	Oil	No.
Nervous tension	bergamot	4	camomile	9	benzoin	4
			camphor	5	jasmine	7
			cypress	4	neroli	5
			geranium	6	patchouli	5
			lavender	4	rose	7
			marjoram	5	sandalwood	5
			melissa	4	ylang-ylang	6
Neuralgia	eucalyptus	8	camomile	9		
			geranium	6		
			peppermint	7		
Nose bleed			cypress	4	frankincense	7
Obesity			fennel	6	patchouli	5
			juniper	5		
Oedema			juniper	5	patchouli	5
Pre-menstrual tension	clary-sage	5	camomile	9	neroli	5
			geranium	6	rose	7
			lavender	4		
			melissa	4		
Rheumatism (including rheumatoid arthritis)						
(general)	eucalyptus	8	cypress	4	benzoin	4
			hyssop	6		
			juniper	5		
			lavender	4		
			rosemary	6		
(local)	eucalyptus	8	camomile	9		
			camphor	5		
			lavender	4		
			rosemary	6		
Shock			camphor	5	neroli	5
			melissa	4		
			peppermint	7		

cont'd

Problem	Top notes	Odour intensity	Middle notes	Odour intensity	Base notes	Odour intensity
Sinus	eucalyptus	8	lavender	4		
			peppermint	7		
Sprains	eucalyptus	8	camphor	5		
			lavender	4		
			rosemary	6		
Sunstroke			lavender	4		
Skin						
acne	bergamot	4	camphor	5	cedarwood	4
			juniper	5	sandalwood	5
			lavender	4		
boils (local)	clary-sage	5	camomile	9		
			lavender	4		
chapped			camomile	9	benzoin	4
			geranium	6	patchouli	5
					rose	7
					sandalwood	5
Skin						
dermatitis			camomile	9	benzoin	4
			hyssop	6		
			geranium	6		
			juniper	5		
			lavender	4		
			peppermint	7		
dry			camomile	9		
			lavender	4		
			geranium	6		
eczema	bergamot	4	camomile	9		
			camphor	5		
			hyssop	6		
			juniper	5		
			lavender	4		

Condition	Oils (drops)
herpes	bergamot 4, eucalyptus 8, clary-sage 5 · cypress 4, lavender 4, myrrh 7 · benzoin 4, frankincense 7, myrrh 7, neroli 5, patchouli 5, rose 7
mature	bergamot 4, lemon 7 · cedarwood 4, ylang-ylang 6
Skin oily	bergamot 4, lemon 7 · camphor 5, cypress 4, geranium 6, juniper 5, lavender 4
psoriasis	bergamot 4 · lavender 4
regenerating & rejuvenating	lemon 7 · lavender 4, melissa 4 · frankincense 7, jasmine 7, myrrh 7, neroli 5, patchouli 5, jasmine 7, neroli 5, rose 7
sensitive	camomile 9
Throat infections	clary 5, euclyptus 8 · geranium 6, lavender 4
Tonsilitis	bergamot 4
Toothache	camomile 9, camphor 5, peppermint 7
Varicose veins (local)	cypress 4

Mineral oil is not effective as it has low penetration power, thereby restricting the essential oil molecules entering the skin.

The formulae must suit the client's physical and mental condition. In general terms 3 per cent dilution of the essential oil/s with a carrier oil is used. As there is a variance in density between a carrier oil and the essential oil, an approximate 1 per cent dilution would be one drop of essential oil to 4 ml of carrier oil.

Storage of oils

They should be kept in dark-coloured air-tight glass bottles (never use plastic) and stored in a cool, dark and dry atmosphere.

Types of massage used for aromatherapy

The main purposes of the massage are:

1. to aid oil penetration;
2. to stimulate generally;
3. for relaxation;
4. to treat localised areas;
5. to treat by way of nerve supply reflexes;
6. to treat by way of meridians.

Massage techniques incorporate the best features of five types of massage:

Swedish massage   using effleurage which influences oil absorption and circulation.

Neuro-muscular massage using friction, vibration and pressure influencing the nerve pathways and muscles. For this purpose it is useful to know that reflex zones correspond to the sympathetic nervous system and are divided into cervical (C), thoracic (T), lumbar (L) and sacral (S) ganglia. Fibres pass from the ganglia to form plexuses from which nerves radiate to supply not only muscles but various internal organs of the body. Fig. 15.2(a) denotes the zones with a brief résumé of the corresponding areas. Therefore by applying pressure on either side of the spine, the ganglia are stimulated and impulses are sent to the relevant internal organ or area. The therapist can gauge the various pressures required by practising these on a weighing machine so that undue pressure is not used.

There are also zones on the face and as seen in Fig. 15.2(b) and pressure made on certain areas will also relate to organs in the body, e.g. the zone above the maxillae bone corresponds to the digestive system.

Connective tissue massage and lymphatic drainage massage   of the body, if these are known, are useful when performing aromatherapy massage.

Table 15.3 Oils to be used with caution

To avoid the risk of skin irritation, skin sensitisation or general toxicity it is inadvisable to use the following oils for any treatments.

Bitter almond,
Boldo leaf,
Horseradish,
Mugwort,
Pennyroyal,
Rue,
Sassafras ,
Southernwood,
Tansy,
Thuya (except when used in minute quantities to cure warts)
Wormwood.

It is inadvisable to use the following on the skin:

Cassia,
Cinnamon bark,
Clove,
Fennel (bitter),
Origanum,
Savory.

The following oils should be used with caution on the skin:

All citrus oils,
Angelica root,
Aniseed,
Basil,
Bergamot,
Caraway,
Cumin,
Verbena,
Ylang Ylang.

The following oils should not be used during pregnancy by either therapist or client:

Basil,
Cinnamon,
Hyssop,
Myrrh,
Origanum,
Pennyroyal,
Sage,
Savory,
Sweet majoram,
Tarragon,
Thyme.

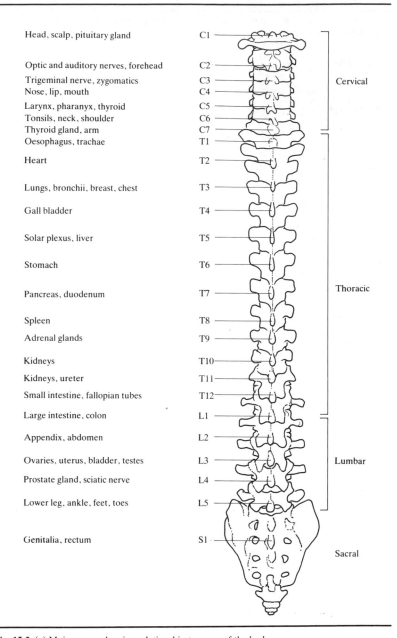

Head, scalp, pituitary gland	C1	
Optic and auditory nerves, forehead	C2	
Trigeminal nerve, zygomatics	C3	Cervical
Nose, lip, mouth	C4	
Larynx, pharanyx, thyroid	C5	
Tonsils, neck, shoulder	C6	
Thyroid gland, arm	C7	
Oesophagus, trachae	T1	
Heart	T2	
Lungs, bronchii, breast, chest	T3	
Gall bladder	T4	
Solar plexus, liver	T5	
Stomach	T6	
Pancreas, duodenum	T7	Thoracic
Spleen	T8	
Adrenal glands	T9	
Kidneys	T10	
Kidneys, ureter	T11	
Small intestine, fallopian tubes	T12	
Large intestine, colon	L1	
Appendix, abdomen	L2	
Ovaries, uterus, bladder, testes	L3	Lumbar
Prostate gland, sciatic nerve	L4	
Lower leg, ankle, feet, toes	L5	
Genitalia, rectum	S1	Sacral

Fig. 15.2 (a) Major zones showing relationship to areas of the body

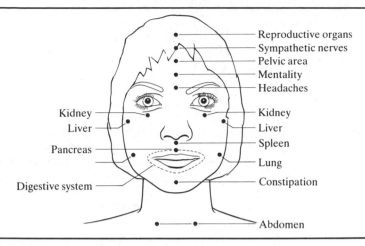

Fig. 15.2 (b) Zones of the face

Shiatsu massage using finger pressure influences the harmonious flow of energy through the body using the Yin and Yang energy meridians and certain points of Shiatsu acupressure. It is assumed that most students will have very little knowledge of this subject; therefore only the basic pressure points are shown on Fig. 15.3 and 15.4.

Yin meridians flow up the body, i.e. from the feet to the head and also the arms if these are held above the head. Yang meridians flow down the body, i.e. from the head to the feet and again the arms if held above the head (from the fingers to the shoulders). Some of these meridians are shown in Figs 15.5(a) and 15.5(b).

All meridian lines connect with the organs of the body as well as other systems, physical and mental. In aromatherapy we are mainly concerned with the bladder meridian and the governing vessel. The latter (as seen in Fig. 15.5b) runs up the centre of the back to the top of the head and the bladder meridian has two tracks on either side of the spine.

Clients also come into the general category of Yin or Yang type pattern of behaviour:

Yin	*Yang*
Slender	Well-made
Weak	Strong
Listless	Active

However, the interwoven complexity of Yin and Yang would apply if a well-made client was listless. When deciding the type of massage, the predominant aspect of the client must be considered first. For a Yin-type client, the massage must be performed in the direction of the meridian flow (i.e. up the Yin meridian and down the Yang meridian). The opposite would apply if the client was predominantly Yang (i.e. against the meridian flow, down the Yin meridians and up the Yang meridians).

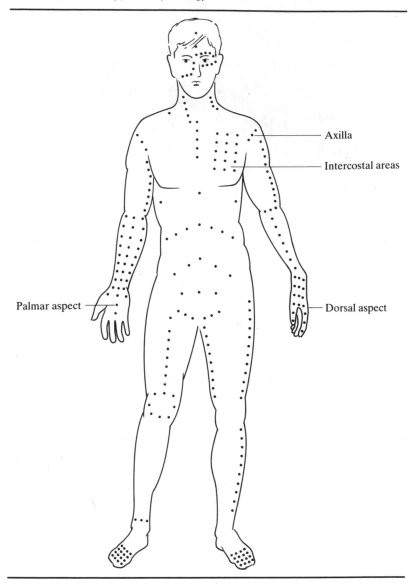

Fig. 15.3 Basic Shiatsu pressure points – anterior view

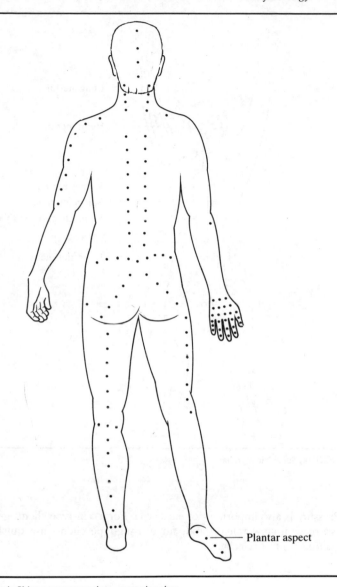

Plantar aspect

Fig. 15.4 Basic Shiatsu pressure points – posterior view

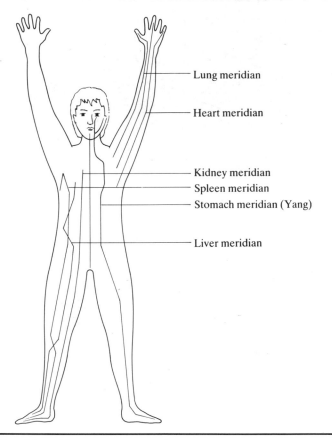

Fig. 15.5 (a) Some Yin meridians

Pressure is also important for each type. For a Yin-type client, give gentle pressure with slow release and, for a Yang-type client, use quick, strong pressure with fast release.

Reflexology

Reflexology is a zone therapy dealing with the principle that there are reflexes in the feet relating to each organ and all parts of the body. Reflexology is generally used as a diagnostic check before giving an aromatherapy massage. Reflexology governs a reflex action of an organ, muscle or gland reached by an energy current initiated by a stimulus. Unlike nerves these

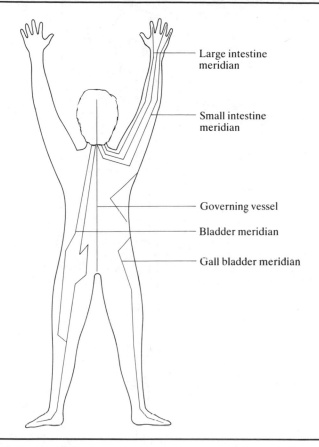

Large intestine
meridian

Small intestine
meridian

Governing vessel

Bladder meridian

Gall bladder meridian

Fig 15.5 (b) Some Yang meridians

energy reflexes do not cross over the spinal column (see Fig. 15.6). There are cross reflexes and these run from the shoulders to the hips, elbows to the knees and from the hands to the feet.

Reflexology can:

● remove waste deposits;
● balance polarity;
● remove congestion and blockages from the energy pathways;
● improve circulation;
● relax the body and mind, so relieving stress and tension.

It will be seen from Fig. 15.7 that the feet resemble the body, i.e. the big toes are the head, the balls of the feet are the shoulders and the arch of the feet resembles the curve of the spine. Organs in the lower part of the body are found in the lower part of the feet and those above the waist are found above the 'waist' of the feet.

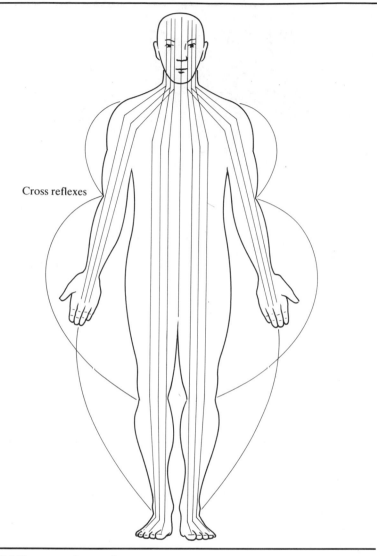

Fig. 15.6 The zones and cross reflexes

For diagnostic purposes the pressure applied to the reflex points is only sufficient to explore if there are any disorders present. If there is a blockage or congestion in the energy channels, acid crystals, waste or unused calcium deposits form in the nerve endings of the feet. When pressure is applied, the client may experience an unpleasant feeling, from tenderness to a grittiness or even to a sharp knife-like pain. It is therefore important to watch the client's face for any reaction.

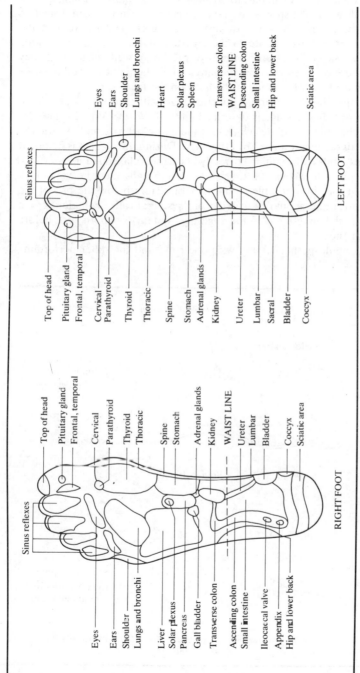

Fig. 15.7 Reflexology chart – plantar aspect of foot

RIGHT FOOT

Sinus reflexes

Top of head
Pituitary gland
Frontal, temporal
Cervical
Parathyroid
Thyroid
Thoracic
Spine
Stomach
Adrenal glands
Kidney
WAIST LINE
Ureter
Lumbar
Bladder
Coccyx
Sciatic area

Eyes
Ears
Shoulder
Lungs and bronchi
Liver
Solar plexus
Pancreas
Gall bladder
Transverse colon
Ascending colon
Small intestine
Ileocaecal valve
Appendix
Hip and lower back

LEFT FOOT

Sinus reflexes

Eyes
Ears
Shoulder
Lungs and bronchi
Heart
Solar plexus
Spleen
Transverse colon
WAIST LINE
Descending colon
Small intestine
Hip and lower back
Sciatic area

Top of head
Pituitary gland
Frontal, temporal
Cervical
Parathyroid
Thyroid
Thoracic
Spine
Stomach
Adrenal glands
Kidney
Ureter
Lumbar
Sacral
Bladder
Coccyx

The reflexes are very small but, to do any good, they must be found and, as pain is not always in the specific area diagnosed, i.e. referred pain, travel up and down the zones carefully. For instance, if there is a disorder in the stomach area it may well relate to the digestive system, so the entire area should be massaged. Pressure in the eye area may well relate to kidney problems, therefore pressure over the latter reflex should be carried out. See Figs. 15.7 and 15.8 for the areas of the body on the feet.

To relax the client, perform a foot massage with a little oil or talcum powder (part of this massage is described under *Pedicure*, Vol. 1 Chap. 24) by rotating the ankles and toes clockwise and anti-clockwise and use friction on the soles of the feet followed by effleurage. During this stage it is helpful if the client responds by breathing correctly in a slow, relaxed manner.

To carry out reflexology the therapist's thumb nails must be very short (especially at the side) and filed back to about 2 mm below the pad of the thumb. The routine should be carried out systematically, completing one system (with the exception of the digestive system) on both feet before beginning the next.

The foot should be held firmly with one hand and the other performing

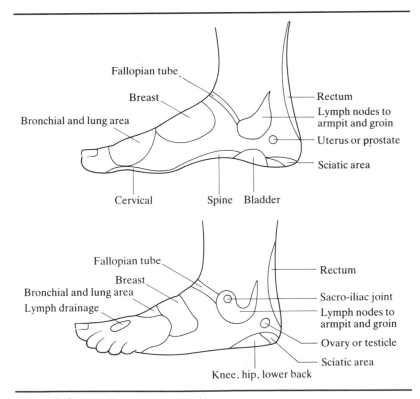

Fig. 15.8 Reflexology chart – dorsal aspect of foot

pressure with the ball of the thumb with the thumb bent at right angles. The side of the thumb may be used for a small area where it is placed on the reflex and is slightly rotated without moving over the skin.

Three photographs are given to show the position of the hands, but the therapist should be able to follow the pressure points from the diagrams of the feet.

Nervous system

Commence at the solar plexus which is just under the ball of the foot as this pressure helps to relax nervous tension (see Fig. 15.9). Move down to the sciatic area and begin pressure across the heel of the foot.

Endocrine glands

The lower part of the big toe represents the pituitary gland. Massage over this reflex may benefit disorders which involve other endocrine glands. The parathyroid and thyroid glands are near the medial aspect of the soles of the feet. The reflex for the sex gland is just under the cushion of the 4th toe. The reflex for the adrenal gland is just superior to the kidney.

Sinuses, eye and ear

Reflexes for the sinuses are in the centre of the cushion in each toe; for the eyes they are just below the neck of the 2nd and 3rd toe; and for the ears, just below the neck of the 4th and 5th toe. Massage here will relieve cold symptoms and catarrh.

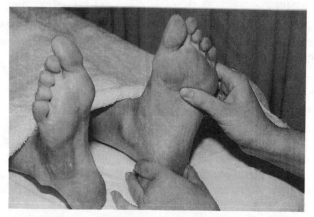

Fig. 15.9 Reflexology – holding the foot with thumb pressure for the solar plexus

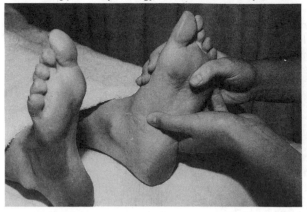

Fig. 15.10 Reflexology – for the spine, pressure on median curve of the foot

Bones and muscular system

For the spine, pressure should be made from the cervical to the coccyx all the way down the median curve of the foot (see Fig. 15.10).

For the neck and shoulder area pressure is applied all round the big toe for the former and for the latter, pressure is applied to the lateral side of the foot just below the neck of the little toe and the cervical area. This will relieve tension in the area.

The reflex for the hip, knee and lower back can be found on the lateral side of the foot above the sciatic area and also just superior to the reflex for the bladder on the medial side of the foot.

Respiratory system

Pressure points for the lungs and bronchi are in the centre of the ball of the foot. They can also be found on the anterior aspect of the foot just below the base of the toes.

Excretory system

This includes the bladder, ureter, kidneys and rectum. The reflex for the bladder will be found on the medial side of the foot just below the lumbar/sacral area. The ureter is a narrow area from the bladder up to the kidney and the use of the side of the thumb is helpful to pin-point this. The kidney reflex is above this and pressure here should not be excessive. The rectum can be found either side of the tendon calcaneum.

Digestive system

For this system it is suggested that you commence on the liver reflex, which is the large area on the lateral side of the right foot. Move down to the gall bladder which lies on the medial lower edge of the liver. As the entrance of the stomach is on the medial side of the right foot, begin your pressure there before moving to the left foot for most of the stomach. The use of the side of the thumb is helpful to pin-point this area.

The small intestine is situated below the waist of both feet from the middle to the median edge. Exert pressure on the client's right foot first and then move over to the left foot.

Remember, as the client is facing you her right foot will be on your left and vice-versa.

The appendix, ileocaecal valve and ascending colon reflexes will be found at the lower lateral edge of the right foot. Work carefully up the colon and just before the waist of the foot move along the transverse colon. Cross to the left foot and continue along the transverse colon and down the descending colon.

Reproductive system

The ovaries or testicles lie on the anterior lateral side of the foot between the lateral melleolus and the achilles tendon (tendon calcaneum).

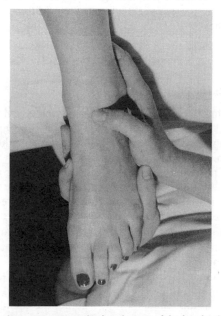

Fig. 15.11 Reflexology – pressure on the dorsal aspect of the foot for the fallopian tubes

The uterus or prostrate lie on the anterior medial side of the foot below the medial malleolus.

The fallopian tubes stretch across the dorsal aspect of the foot just above the lymph nodes to the groin and armpit (see Fig. 15.11). Reflexes for the breasts are also found on the dorsal aspect of the foot.

Circulatory system

The heart reflex is found on the left foot slightly to the right of the solar plexus.

Lymphatic system

The spleen can be found to the right of the stomach reflex.

Lymph nodes to the groin and armpits are found just below the lateral malleolus and those for the cervical area lie between the base of the first and second toes on the anterior aspect of the foot.

When you have completed the diagnosis return to the reflexes which showed a small problem area. This will help you to decide on the essential oils that you should now use.

Do remember that many reflexes overlap and sometimes it is difficult to assess the exact nature of the problem. Further in-depth study of reflexology will be needed to be absolutely certain for any curative sessions.

Use effleurage movements over the entire feet, finishing with pressure on the solar plexus reflexes.

Consultation with the client

Talking and listening to clients is paramount. Without prying into personal affairs, a great deal can be learnt about their personality, general health and life-style. For example, do they have a sedentary occupation or lead a full and active life? Do they drive a car long distances? Do they require concentration to operate machinery or do they suffer from stress and frustration? Stress manifests itself in various ways from running a home and coping with children to a managerial-executive position demanding responsibility and decisions, or even both.

It is important to carry out a diagnosis prior to any treatment. A record card should be kept and Fig. 15.12 shows a specimen card which can be adapted to your requirements.

The diagnosis in detail should consider the following:

Height and weight   as this will determine whether the client is over or under weight.

Name: ....   Date: ....

Address: ....

....

Telephone No: ....

Occupation: (if known)   ....

Medical history: ....

....

Medication presently taken: ....

....

Name of Doctor: (if necessary)   ....

Address: ....

Telephone No: ....

Signature of Client: ....

Diagnosis:

    Height   ....

    Weight   ....

    Posture   ....

    Muscle tone   ....

    Circulation   ....

Lymphatic system   ....

Skin tone & colour of skin   ....

Essential oils chosen   ....

....

Fig. 15.12 Specimen record card

Posture   as explained in Chapter 2, should be taken into consideration.

Muscle tone   can be felt by placing the client in a prone position on the plinth and running the hands over the body. Note whether the muscles are tensed or relaxed, i.e. are they tender or do they feel like chords? If nodules are present on muscles, this would probably indicate stress or a fibrotic condition. If there is a lack of elasticity, this usually denotes lack of use, tiredness or fatigue.

Circulation   can be observed in many ways. Cold hands and feet, chilblains, thread or varicose veins in the legs all point to poor circulation. By running the side of the thumb-nail down the spine, circulation can be seen by the colour remaining. Pinking would suggest general good circulation but any white patches would indicate local poor circulation which would affect the organs the nerves supply.

When the client is in a supine position look at the face to see if there are any congested areas, i.e. nose and chin.

Use light pressure over the abdomen to check for any tenderness or tension which may arise from constipation or gynaecological problems.

The lymphatic system   if working well, the lymph will circulate freely and there will be no evidence of oedema or cellulite. Therefore note if the client has swollen ankles, water retention (e.g. rings very tight on the fingers) and/ or the body tissues are spongy.

The skin tone   should be recorded, where it is slack, tight or congested. If it has a goose-flesh effect it may be an indication that there is an excessive amount of acidity in the system.

The colour of the skin   should be observed as this can reveal a great deal about your client.

A pale skin will denote a tendency to anaemia and/or low blood pressure. Flushed facial skin may signal high blood pressure. A yellowish sallow skin may indicate toxicity, probably due to poor digestion affecting the liver, stomach or bowels. Grey skins often indicate nervous exhaustion or excess fatigue.

When you have treated your client make a note of any area that has become reddened or 'blotched'. Discolouration can often point to problems in corresponding organs. This may result in a different selection of essential oils at the next treatment.

Contra-indications to aromatherapy massage

● abnormal temperature;
● advanced heart condition;

severe asthma;

recent fracture and recent scar tissue;

advanced cancer condition;

varicose veins;

post-operative condition or if the client is receiving medical treatment (unless the doctor is consulted and agrees the massage may be given);

hyperthyroid condition;

immediately following an inoculation;

avoid an area where there is inflammation, infection, broken skin or bruises;

pregnancy (unless you have sound knowledge of the specific treatment);

two days before and the first two days of menstruation.

It is also unwise to give aromatherapy if the client is very hungry or has just eaten a heavy meal. Sport of any kind can make a client tired, muscles tense and it would be preferable to leave the aromatherapy for at least an hour and advise the client to rest.

Suggested aromatherapy massage procedure

Prepare the room and the couch and warm the client, preferably with infra-red, and mix the oils to be used.

1. Lie client on the abdomen and wrap up legs. Have modesty towels and forehead pillow (or folded towel) to hand.
2. Slowly, with appropriate oil, effleurage entire back/buttock area.
3. Place left hand on occipital lobe and leave there.
4. Place right hand flat on 5th thoracic ganglia for a few seconds, lift slowly and repeat on 10th thoracic and finally on the 2nd/3rd lumbar.
5. Slide right hand up erector spinae to cranium and slide both hands down to sacro-coccyx joint.
6. With reinforced hand (i.e. one hand over the other to give firm pressure) stroke up each side of the erector spinae taking the hand over the scapula followed by light pressure down to the sacro-coccyx joint (times 3).
7. Slide both hands up lower erector spinae and fan out over right and left iliac crest, pushing slightly towards the feet. Return hands to sacro-coccyx joint (times 3).
8. Using both thumbs apply pressure around sacro-coccyx area (as a triangle) (times 3).
9. Use pressure movements with thumbs from the sacrum following the iliac crest and slide hands back to sacrum (times 3).
10. Again use pressure movements from sacrum to sciatic plexus, rest hands flat on area, effleurage area and return to sacrum (times 3).
11. Apply pressure with thumbs from lumbar-sacral plexus L4–S3 following sciatic nerve to buttocks, slide hands back (times 3).
12. Apply pressure with thumbs from L3–L4 to buttocks and Lat. femoral cutaneous nerve, slide hands back (times 3).

13. Effleurage area and cover the buttocks with a towel.
14. With thumbs apply pressure and sliding movements up either side of the erector spinae from L5 to C3. Turn the thumbs to face each other approximately 2 cm from the spinal column on one side. Press firmly down with the thumbs and release. Move the lower thumb down a full thumb's length, then slide other thumb to meet the former using pressure all the time down to L5. Repeat these movements on the other side of the spinal column.
15. Circles for the back. With both hands stroke firmly up the back, over the scapula and make circles, finishing a little lower on the upper thoracic area. Make another circle over this area and continue making circles down the back, finishing at the lumbar area.
16. Stroke firmly with both hands (either side of the spinal column) from L5 to the scapula, returning lightly to the L5. Again from the L5 stroke firmly to the axillae, returning lightly to L4. From here firm strokes to T10 returning again to L4.
17. To loosen the tissue with both hands over the entire back (but being careful not to pinch), move the hands up one side of the spinal column to the trapezius. Turn the hands horizontally (fingers pointing outward) and move the lower hand about 3–4 in. (9 cm) down. Push the fingers of both hands together (letting the thumbs overlap) (see Fig. 15.13) and quickly release. Move the hands down and repeat towards the axillae. This is often called 'raking' the back. Continue with these movements (about five in total) down to the lumbar area. Repeat these movements on the other side of the spinal column.
18. Place one hand over the other and slide hands up to T1 (with fingers pointing outwards) apply firm pressure and push fingers out to the axillae along the thoracic nerve pathways. Move the hands down about 1 in. (2.5 cm) and repeat to L1. Move the fingers to the other side of the spinal column and repeat these movements.
19. From the top of the pelvic girdle use fanning movements to the axillae

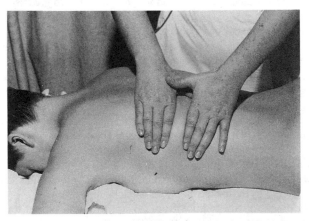

Fig. 15.13 Aromatherapy – 'raking' the back

and over the scapula, i.e. using alternate hands with open fingers and as the first hand moves up the body it also goes sideways like a fan and the second hand follows. Repeat on the other side of the back and return to L4 (see Figs. 15.14(a) and 15.14(b)).

20. Slide hand from lumbar to kidney area and rest. Slide both hands to brachial plexus and rest, then up to trapezius and rest. Return hands to L4. Effleurage kidney area.

21. Slide hands to thoracic area with light pressure use thumbs between intercostal spaces (times 3). Effleurage the area and return to L4.

22. Use firm pressure (with either thumb or two fingers) either side of the spinal column from L4 to C3 and slide hands lightly and slowly down to L4 (times 3).

23. Slide one hand up to the thoracic area and with the other cover the client with a towel. Slide both hands up to cervical plexus across the trapezius, over the acromion process and as the hands are drawn back slightly, pull on the trapezius to C3 (times 3).

24. Slide hands to cervical ganglia and use deep thumb pressures along trapezius, slide hands back (times 3).

25. Stand at the head of the client (place forehead on pillow or towel) and from the trapezius use firm pressure up sternocleidomastoid to temporal bone. Slide hands back to trapezius (times 3).

26. Hold right side of head with left hand. With right thumb (or first two fingers) apply pressure from cervical ganglia to postauricular node, temporal and occipital bone (vagus nerve) and cranial fissure.

27. Repeat on left side of head (as step 26).

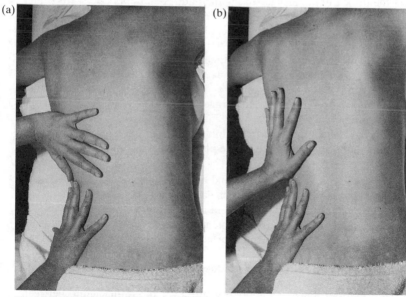

Fig. 15.14 (a) Aromatherapy – fanning movements
(b) Aromatherapy – fanning movements

28. Effleurage scapula/trapezius/sternocleidomastoid ending with light pressure on the cranium (times 3).
29. Make client comfortable again and cover entire back area and unwrap left leg.
30. Apply oil, effleurage from plantar surface of the foot to gluteal ridge (times 3).
31. Rest left hand on plantar surface of foot, slide right hand up and rest on popliteal space, slide up to gluteal ridge, apply pressure and slide hand down to achilles tendon.
32. Apply thumb pressure along achilles tendon, calcaneum and talus. Effleurage (times 3).
33. Deep effleurage to gluteal ridge. Slide hands back to the popliteal space and use thumb pressures up the leg covering (a) biceps femoris, vastus lateralis to gluteus maximus; (b) biceps femoris, semitendinosus; and (c) gracillus, abductor magnus muscles.
34. Apply thumb pressures down sciatic nerve to popliteal space.
35. Effleurage area (times 3).
36. Rest hand on popliteal space, then perform thumb pressures on tibial nerve to achilles tendon.
37. Slide hands back to popliteal space and use thumb pressures along peroneal nerve to achilles tendon.
38. Effleurage lower leg, finishing with pressure on the achilles tendon and plantar surface (times 3).
39. Cover up left leg and repeat steps 30–38 for right leg.
40. Turn client on to her back, cover well, leaving right leg uncovered.
41. Effleurage from phalanges to inguinal nodes and apply pressure (times 3).
42. Slide hands to inguinal nodes, apply pressure and slide hands down femoral nerve with light pressure to patella.
43. Thumb pressure around patella (times 3).
44. Apply pressure to the peroneal nerve down to the retinaculum.
45. Slide hands back to the patella and apply pressure to the saphenous nerve to the retinaculum. Effleurage (times 3). Place a towel over the area but leave the foot free.
46. Turn the client's foot upwards. Hold the foot in the hand and using the thumb only, apply pressure on the plantar aspect, commencing at:

    (a) big toe, i.e. the top, middle and base;
    (b) in between the base of each phalange;
    (c) down the lateral side of the foot to the middle of the calcaneum;
    (d) continue slow pressure movements from the centre of the calcaneum to the middle of the plantar surface and out to the median side of the foot;
    (e) give firm pressure over the kidney and solar plexus reflexes.

47. Turn the foot down and apply pressure over the retinaculum, between each metatarsal and to the top of the phalange.

48. Effleurage the entire foot and finish with final pressure at the solar plexus reflex (times 3).
49. Cover right foot and uncover left leg. Repeat 41–46c. Apply pressure from the median side of the foot to the centre and down to the middle of the calcaneum. Repeat 46e–48.
50. Wrap the client and uncover left arm. Apply oil to hand and arm and effleurage (times 3).
51. Palm facing upward, use thumb pressure movements from the carpus to the axillae, covering ulna and median nerves. Apply pressure on the axillary nodes and slide hand down to carpus (times 3).
52. Repeat movements from the carpus to suprascapular nerve, covering the radial and median nerves. Apply gentle pressure and slide hand back to carpus (times 3).
53. Firm pressure over the palmar surface of the hand.
54. Turn hand over and effleurage anterior side of arm, carpus to deltoid. Apply pressure covering all nerve plexuses, i.e. radial, median and ulna, followed by effleurage.
55. Take hand, apply pressure to carpus, each metacarpal and phalange and effleurage to phalange tips.
56. Cover arm and repeat 50–55 for right arm.
57. Unwrap for abdomen, apply oil and effleurage (times 3).
58. Slide hands up the rectus abdominus to the sternum; let the fingers overlap, then separate and pull the hands down and out towards the waist. Apply gentle pressure, turn the hands and following the external abdominal oblique muscles, lift the tissues upwards and pull the hands down and inwards along the iliac crest to the pubis (times 3).
59. Starting at the lower abdomen (at the hypogastric plexus), use light pressure with thumbs from either side of the pubis over the iliac crest, slide hands back (times 3).
60. For the mid-abdomen, starting at the rectus abdominus (or mesenteric plexus), use light pressure to the external oblique muscles and slide hands back (times 3).
61. Move hands up to the coeliac (or solar) plexus, use light pressure through the intercostal spaces to the latissimus dorsi and slide hands back (times 2). Use the ulna side of each hand and alternately stroke down the right and left borders of the rib cage.
62. Slide the hands along the right external oblique muscle towards the latissimus dorsi. Kneading can be performed or the muscles lifted and squeezed towards the lateral side of the body. Hands can continue gentle kneading across the abdomen to the left external oblique muscle where kneading or lifting can be repeated.
63. Slide hands down to the ascending colon, use light pressure up the colon across the transverse colon and down the descending colon. Always slide hands across the bladder (times 3).
64. Effleurage abdomen and finish at the coeliac plexus with light pressure.
65. Cover client well with towel resting on the breasts.
66. Effleurage area from the sternum including the trapezius.

67. Make pressure points from either side of the sternum up to the clavicle. Slide hands back to the sternum (times 3).
68. Firm pressure points beneath the clavicle to the axillae. Slide hands back and repeat times 3.

To complete the aromatherapy massage the following procedure is suggested for the face.

It may be appropriate to change the oil for the face and therefore the hands must be washed. Ensure that the client's body is covered with towels and blanket to retain warmth. Stand at the head of the couch for this massage.

69. Slide the hands to pectoralis major, over deltoids. Use thumb pressure over acromion process, along trapezius to sternocleidomastoid (times 3).
70. Again slide hands to the pectorals, over deltoid and acromion process and move to the erector spinae. Apply pressure to C7, C5 and C2 and very slightly stretch the neck.
71. Slide hands back to the pectorals and over deltoid. Use very slow, firm pressure along the trapezius to the base of the cranium.
72. Slide the hands down the trapezius to the clavicle and use firm pressure movements above the clavicle to the sternum. Slide hands b ick to the trapezius and repeat the thumb pressures (times 3).
73. Effleurage the neck area and slide the hands to the temporalis. Make firm pressure with the first two fingers all along the hairline and back to the temporalis.
74. Spread the fingers at the hairline and move them on to the scalp. Maintaining contact with the skin, perform friction massage movements all over the scalp, changing the position of the fingers until all the scalp has had friction massage (see Fig. 15.15). Finish by sliding hands down the sternocleidomastoid muscle.
75. Perform gently upward effleurage movements over the neck and face with both hands. Use ring fingers to perform circular movements around the eyes finishing at the temples.
76. Leave the fingers at the temporalis and place thumbs, one on top of the other, on the procerus and make pressure and release movements here. Move the thumbs up (about the width of the thumb) and repeat the thumb pressure and release; continue in this way up the frontalis to the hairline and then stroke the area with alternate thumbs.
77. Return the thumbs to the procerus and apply pressure and release along the corrugator to the temporalis. Slide the thumbs back to the centre of the frontalis and use pressure and release back to the temporalis, but each time move a thumb's width up the frontalis until the whole area has been covered. Again make thumb circles to stroke the entire frontalis (see Fig. 15.16).
78. Leave the thumbs on the frontalis and use the second and third fingers to apply pressure and release from the nasalis over the zygomatics, thereby draining the sinus area. Move the fingers down (about the width of one finger) and repeat the pressure and release movement under the zygomatics (times 3).

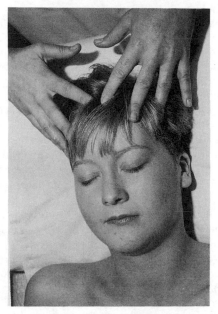

Fig. 15.15 Aromatherapy – friction massage movements over the scalp from the hairline

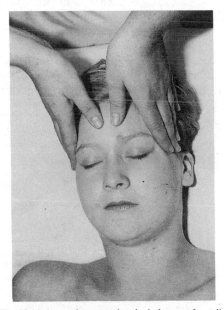

Fig. 15.16 Aromatherapy – thumb circles over frontalis

79. Release the thumbs and, using two fingers, apply pressure and release over the buccinator, risorius, orbicularis oris finishing at the mentalis (times 3).
80. Slide the fingers under the mandible and apply pressure and release along towards the temporomandibular joint. Slide the fingers back to the centre of the mandible (times 3).
81. Slide the fingers on to the mandible and place the index fingers on the superior orbicularis oris and the second and third fingers (of both hands) on the inferior orbicularis oris and pull gently out and up towards the temporalis (times 3).
82. Slide hands down to the superior orbicularis oris and with the ring finger of the right hand apply pressure and release up the right side of the nasalis to the procerus. Repeat with the left ring finger on the left side of the nasalis to the procerus.
83. With both ring fingers apply very gentle pressure and release all round the orbicularis oculi (times 3). Finish with pressure and slightly lifting the corrugator to the temporalis.
84. Slide hands down to the clavicle and effleurage the entire neck and face (times 3). Each sequence should be lighter than the former, finishing with very light pressure on the temporalis.
85. Complete the wrapping of the client and leave to rest. Take this time to make any notes or remarks on the client's record card/sheet.

The client should be given a glass of water to drink and advised to avoid a bath or shower for at least 6–8 hours after the massage to ensure full absorption of the essential oils.

Aromatherapy is a complex subject and students are advised to widen their knowledge by reading the many books and articles written (including the history and origin of this ancient art which is not covered in this chapter), and to include a study of Shiatsu massage to understand the subject further. Where training is concerned, there are courses available for therapists. Several techniques exist, as standardisation of these is difficult, but basically it is a matter of individual interpretation together with an affinity with the oils used.

Chapter 16

First-aid

To have some knowledge of this subject does help when the unexpected happens in the salon. The Red Cross and St John's Ambulance run courses which are invaluable. The following are a few symptoms or conditions which you may come across together with immediate first-aid suggestions.

Artificial respiration (or the kiss of life)

This is a method of forcing air into and out of the lungs to start breathing in a person whose breathing has stopped which may happen following an electric shock, choking or a heart attack. There are two main methods, by external chest compression and/or mouth-to-mouth respiration. Compression should only be used by those trained in first aid.

A person who has stopped breathing will die within minutes, therefore it is important to force air into the lungs as quickly as possible. To see if someone is breathing, listen at the mouth and nose and look to see if the chest is moving. Check the pulse at carotid artery by placing your fingers in the hollows of the neck between the Adam's Apple and the muscle at the side.

First of all, open the airway by lying the person flat on his/her back and tilt the head back by lifting under the neck with one hand and pressing the forehead down with the other hand.

To ensure that the tongue is not blocking the opening to the trachea take your hand from the neck and lift the chin upwards.

Turn the head to one side and clear the mouth of any debris (i.e. saliva or vomit which may have collected) by sweeping inside it with two fingers.

If the person is still not breathing, turn the head back, lift up the chin and pinch the nose with your finger and thumb of one hand.

Seal your lips around the person's open mouth and give four quick breaths.

Remove your mouth and check the pulse at the neck and see if the chest is moving. If breathing has not recommenced, replace your mouth and begin breathing into the person at a normal rate until breathing is resumed or medical assistance arrives (see Figs. 16.1 to 16.5).

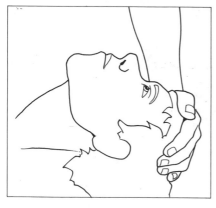

Fig. 16.1 Artificial respiration – lift head back

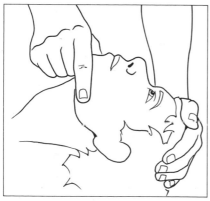

Fig. 16.2 Artificial respiration – lift up chin

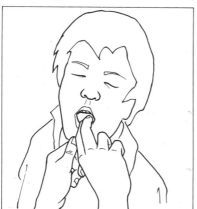

Fig. 16.3 Artificial respiration – clear mouth of any debris

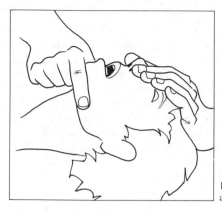

Fig. 16.4 Artificial respiration – lift the chin and pinch the nose

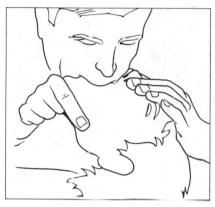

Fig. 16.5 Artificial respiration – seal the mouth with your own lips

Blisters

These can be quite painful but if left alone most will heal within a week, whether or not they burst. Never burst a blister unless the taut skin is causing discomfort as once the skin of a blister is broken bacteria can enter and this increases the risk of infection. However, if the need to burst a blister is absolutely necessary observe the highest hygenic conditions.

1. Wash your hands thoroughly and dry with paper tissues.
2. Wash the blistered area with soapy water with an antiseptic added.
3. Take a fine needle through a flame and let it cool.
4. Do not touch the point of the needle and leave the black sooty appearance. Press the point of the needle gently but firmly into the skin on one side of the blister, just enough to puncture it. Remove the needle and repeat a second puncture on the other side of the blister.
5. Wipe the blister gently with an antiseptic solution and apply an adhesive dressing.

Burns and scalds

Burns are caused by contact with dry heat (fire), electricity, strong chemicals, lighting or the ultra-violet rays of the sun and friction. Scalds are caused by boiling water, steam or hot oils. The treatment for burns and scalds is identical and the depth and area will determine the seriousness. First-degree burns damage the epidermis; second-degree burns damage both the epidermis and dermis and third-degree burns damage the epidermis, dermis and subcutaneous tissue. All but minor burns and scalds should be seen by a doctor.

A superficial burn is extremely painful and appears red, swollen and often blistered. A deep burn may not be so painful as the nerve endings will have been damaged and it will appear grey. This can happen with a galvanic burn. Your initial action is as follows.

1. Remove the person from the source of the heat. If the source is electrical, pull out the plug or switch off the power.
2. Remove any tight clothing and, if the burn is on the hands, remove rings and watch before the area starts to swell.
3. Cool the burn with cold water. If it is a finger or wrist it can be held under a slow running tap for ten minutes. A larger area (i.e. a foot or arm) should be plunged into a bucket of cold water for the same time. You should never apply ointment or lotions, touch the burn or scald or break a blister. Areas like the face or chest that cannot be held under water should be covered by a thick cloth (i.e. towel) soaked in cold water. The cloth should be renewed frequently to prevent its becoming warm and dry. Continue with this process for at least ten minutes and it will quickly relieve pain and reduce the formation of blisters.
4. After cooling, cover the burn or scald with a dry dressing and a loose bandage to hold this in place. Plasters should not be used.
5. Reassure the person concerned and keep her/him warm, giving sips of water to replace lost fluid.

In a salon burns can occur with electrical equipment, i.e. galvanism. Scalds can occur if the facial steamer 'spits' or the water in the steambath container boils due to a faulty thermostat. Hot oil masks and paraffin wax treatments can always be at risk if not carefully watched and tested before applying to the client.

Concussion

This is usually caused by either a blow to the head through accidentally falling and knocking the head against furniture or a heavy fall on to the feet which can shake and disturb the brain. The person may be dazed or suffer a spell of unconsciousness followed by nausea and vomiting.

Lay the person down and cover with a blanket to maintain warmth and seek medical advice.

Cramp

This is a sudden involuntary spasm of muscles which causes acute pain. It can be caused by:

1. insufficient warming-up before an exercise class;
2. chilling during or after exercise, especially swimming;
3. poor muscular co-ordination during exercise;
4. poor circulation;
5. loss of salt and body fluids through sweating, vomiting or diarrhoea.

The spasm can be relieved by stretching the muscles affected and massaging them. For cramp in the hand, straighten the fingers, using gentle force, or spread out the fingers and press down on a surface with the tips of the fingers. For cramp in the calf muscles, ask the client to stand up, straighten the knee and press down at the heel and toes alternately. At the same time the client should lean forward slightly to stretch the calf muscles and you should massage the affected muscles.

If cramp persists for any length of time, it may be due to loss of salt from the body through sweating. You should give the client plenty of water slightly salted, e.g. half a teaspoon of salt to one pint of water.

Cuts

Minor cuts rarely need medical advice and can be treated as follows.

1. Stop the bleeding by pressing on the wound with a clean cloth.
2. Clean the skin around the cut with gauze and lukewarm water with soap or a mild antiseptic. Wipe outwards from the cut, changing the gauze frequently, and ensure the water you are using does not enter the cut.
3. Apply a bandage or plaster to the area.

If the cut is deep the bleeding can usually be stopped by pressing a pad of gauze down on to the wound. This helps to slow the flow of blood and allows the blood to clot. If a limb is involved, raise this higher than the heart to reduce the blood pressure and assist the clotting process. Pressure should be maintained for 5–15 minutes and then bandage firmly. Medical advice should be sought immediately if the blood is flowing with a pumping action as an artery may be damaged, or if the cut is so deep that it may require stitches.

Diabetic coma

In discussions with your clients you will know those who require insulin or drugs to control diabetes. Taking too much insulin or eating too little food can result in hypoglycaemia, an abnormally low level of sugar in the blood.

This can also occur after exercise has burnt up the sugar in the blood. This in turn affects the brain and can lead to a coma. The person concerned would have a rapid pulse, become very pale and sweat profusely. An immediate first-aid reaction would be to supply sugar, i.e. sugar, jam, honey, chocolates or sweet soft drinks.

The opposite condition is hyperglycaemia, a lack of insulin, in which case the face of the person concerned would be flushed with a dry skin, and he or she would be breathing deeply with the breath smelling of acetone (pear drops). Diabetics know when this is happening and will take insulin or medication immediately.

If a diabetic does become unconscious put him or her into the recovery position (explained on pp. 331–332, Figs 16.7–16.10) and get immediate medical assistance.

Drug overdose

Rarely will you come into contact with a client in the salon who has taken an overdose of drugs. You should be aware of the symptoms and these can include difficulty in breathing, vomiting, dilation or contraction of the pupils of the eyes (dark centres), sweating and sometimes becoming unconscious.

An overdose can apply to prescribed medicines as well as to addictive drugs. Seek medical help immediately and while awaiting this, keep the client warm and calm and try to ascertain any information about the drug taken.

Electric shock

Electricity can kill, severely burn or asphyxiate a person. Injuries can occur when equipment is not properly earthed and the extent of the injury will depend on the strength of the charge and how long the person was exposed to it.

An electric shock causes violent contraction of a muscle and the person holding the appliance may not be able to break contact with it. Never touch the person during an electrical accident without first insulating yourself. Immediately turn off the power or wrench the plug from the socket by the flex (just in case the plug itself is at fault). If these options are not possible, insulate yourself by either wearing thick-rubber soled shoes or by standing on a rubber mat or a pile of magazines or newspapers. Move the person away from the appliance, using a wooden chair or a broom, or loop a dry towel around an arm or leg to pull the person free. Send immediately for an ambulance.

Breathing may have stopped due to paralysis of the muscles of respiration or muscles of the heart. Apply artificial respiration and continue until breathing has been restored or help has arrived.

Epileptic fit

Sufferers from epilepsy usually carry an identifying card or bracelet and they usually have a few seconds' warning prior to the attack. This may involve a sensation of noise, taste or smell, or even seeing flashing lights.

There are two types of epileptic fit, the *grand mal* – which involves unconsciousness, convulsions and noisy breathing – or a *petit mal*, involving only momentary loss of consciousness or confusion.

When loss of consciousness occurs it may well be followed by the limbs and neck stiffening and then the whole body being overcome by rhythmic and violent twitching. Do not try to restrain the person; instead, clear a space, remove furniture and try to cushion any fall. Loosen all clothing around the neck and abdomen and place a pillow or something soft under the head. Do not put anything into the mouth or try to open it.

After the attack, keep the person warm but do not give anything to drink until you are quite sure that the person has fully regained consciousness and is alert. If by any chance it takes more than fifteen minutes to do so, or the person has been injured, call an ambulance.

Eye injuries

The most common injury to the eye is a foreign body, such as an eyelash, hair or piece of grit.

Contact lens can become displaced or get stuck to the eyeball and, rather than injure the eye, medical help should be advised.

To remove a foreign body:

1. Turn the client's face up to the light and push the eyelids away from the eyeball with your thumb and forefinger. While you look for the object, request the client to look up and down, right and left. A foreign body in the eye may scratch or damage the cornea and therefore no attempt should be made to remove anything if it is lying on the pupil of the eye. The eye should be covered with a clean pad, i.e. a sterilised pad or the inside of a clean, folded handkerchief kept in place with a bandage, and the person should be taken to the doctor or hospital. However, if the foreign body appears on the whites of the eyes or is on the underside of the eyelid, continue with steps 2 and 3.
2. Rinse the eye out with a small solution of salt in warm water. An eye bath is suitable for this purpose.
3. Alternatively tilt the head backwards, press down the lid with a matchstick and pull up the lid against the matchstick with your finger and thumb. Remove the foreign body with the corner of a clean handkerchief (or gauze). Pull the lashes gently down over the eyeball (see Fig. 16.6).

In a salon there may be preparations which can cause painful irritation of the eyeball (i.e. astringents, eyelash tints, peroxide) if they accidentally enter the

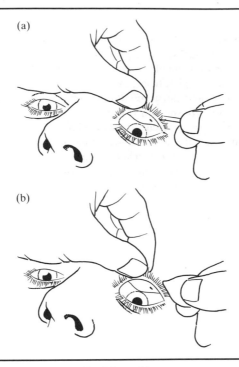

Fig. 16.6 Removing grit on the underside of the eyelid

eye. Should this happen, tilt the client's head to the injured side and gently run cold or lukewarm water, using a small jug, over the eye. You may need to force the eyelid open if it is closed in pain. Dry the face and apply a clean dressing or gauze lightly over the eye.

Fainting and unconsciousness

Fainting is a common cause of brief unconsciousness and is due to the blood supply to the brain being suddenly and temporarily reduced. It can be caused by a hot, stuffy atmosphere, an emotional stimulus, a drop in blood sugar caused by excessive dieting, fatigue or just by standing still for a long time.

A person who feels faint becomes pale, the skin is cold and clammy and beads of sweat often appear on the forehead, neck and hands. Loss of consciousness can sometimes be avoided by lowering the head between the knees and waving smelling salts under the nose. Always make sure there is plenty of fresh air and that clothing is loosened at the neck, chest and abdomen.

For someone who has fainted, lie him or her down on the back, lift the legs above the level of the heart and support them with a chair or something suitable. Turn the head to one side and check that the tongue is forward. Recovery is usually within a few minutes when the person can be seated and given sips of cold water.

Unconsciousness is an abnormal state of lack of response to sensory stimuli resulting from shock, illness or injury. There are three stages of unconsciousness and a person may experience all three or remain in one. These are drowsiness, stupor and coma.

If an unconscious person is not breathing you will need to give artificial respiration and dial 999 for an ambulance. If the unconscious person is breathing he/she should be put into a *recovery position* until medical help arrives, i.e.

1. As with artificial respiration, lie the person on the ground flat on his/her back, clear the mouth of any foreign matter and free the tongue.
2. Turn the person's head towards you. Straighten the near arm and tuck in under the body. Place the other arm across the chest and the far ankle over the near ankle.

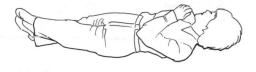

Fig. 16.7 Recovery position

3. Grip the clothing at the far hip, cushion the head with one hand and pull the person towards you.

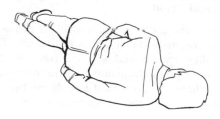

Fig. 16.8 Recovery position

4. Tilt the chin backwards to straighten the throat.
5. Pull the arm out from under the body and bend the other arm to support the upper part of the body. Bend the leg to support the lower part of the body (see Figs. 16.7 to 16.10).

While you wait for medical help, loosen any clothing around the neck, chest

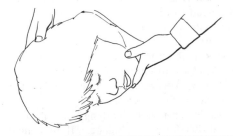

Fig. 16.9 Recovery position

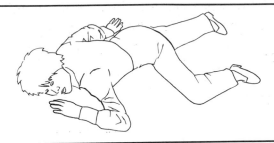

Fig. 16.10 Recovery position

and abdomen. Open a window or door to provide fresh air and stay with the person until medical help arrives.

Fractures, sprains and strains

A *fracture* is a broken or cracked bone which could happen as a result of a fall in a salon. There are two main classifications of fracture. The one you are most likely to encounter is the closed or *simple* fracture where the skin is unbroken. An open or *compound* fracture is where the bone has protruded through the skin or where a deep wound reveals the bone. Although the former cannot be seen, the area will be tender to touch, swollen and often bruised.

Telephone for an ambulance and, while waiting for it to arrive, keep the client warm and comfortable but do not give food or drink just in case an anaesthetic is required later to set the bone.

A *sprain* is the wrenching or twisting of a joint with partial rupture of its ligaments.

A *strain* occurs when a muscle is overstretched or torn.

Treatment for these two injuries are the same. Make a compress of crushed ice-cubes or a simple cold water pad (i.e. a towel soaked in cold water and wrung out) and place this on the area. Keep it wet and cold to help reduce the swelling and leave it in place for about 20–30 minutes. If you are at all concerned that there could be a fracture, medical assistance should be sought.

Grazes

If a client should fall in the street on her way to your salon there may be a graze which you can treat very simply.

1. Wash your hands.
2. Sometimes it is better to let the wound bleed a little to let the blood wash away dirt and bacteria.
3. Any dirt or gravel left around the graze should be removed by washing the area with clean gauze which has been dipped in lukewarm soapy water. Any loose gravel or dirt left in the wound can be removed with gauze soaked in antiseptic or with sterilised tweezers. Always clean the graze from the centre outwards so that infection is not taken into the wound.
4. Dry the area with clean gauze.
5. An adhesive plaster can be applied to a small graze but, for a large graze, use a sterile dressing and fix it in place with either a bandage or sticking plaster. Avoid using cotton wool as the fibres will stick to the wound.
6. If the graze is very dirty, advise the client to seek medical advice.

Heart attacks

The main symptom leading to a heart attack is a severe, crushing pain in the chest, often spreading to the neck and jaw and to one or both arms. The person may suffer giddiness or become breathless and sweat profusely. Shock may follow lapsing into unconsciousness.

If the client is conscious, place him/her on the floor into a half-sitting position with pillows or towels behind the head and shoulders and under the knees. Loosen all tight clothing around the neck, chest and waist and dial 999 for an ambulance. Do not give anything to eat or drink.

If the person becomes unconscious and is not breathing, give artificial respiration. If unconscious but breathing he or she should be put into the recovery position until the ambulance arrives.

Hysterical attacks

These are usually caused by an emotional upset or mental stress. The person concerned usually likes an audience to gain sympathy and attention. It may resemble an epileptic fit if the person concerned shouts or screams, tears at clothing or hair, rolls on the ground or clutches at other people. However genuinely distressed that person may be, it is rare that he or she will come to any harm.

Reassure and try to calm the client, speak gently but firmly and take him/her out of the salon to a quiet area. Never slap an hysterical person, especially an older client who may have a weak heart. Once the attack has subsided, suggest that medical advice be sought.

Nose bleeding

This often happens when a small blood vessel inside the nose is ruptured. It can happen after a bout of sneezing, an attack of hay fever or a nasal infection, and yet it can happen for no apparent reason. Although the blood loss looks great it is rarely very serious and will generally clear up in 5–15 minutes. If this happens in the salon:

1. sit the client down and ensure the clothing around the neck is loose;
2. incline the head slightly forward to help prevent the client swallowing too much blood and use a bowl or towel to catch the drops of blood;
3. ask the client to breathe gently through the mouth and lightly pinch the nostrils closed for 5–10 minutes; this is the time it usually takes for blood to clot;
4. if the bleeding persists you should seek medical assistance.

Poisoning

This rarely happens in a salon as accidental poisoning usually occurs in the home, mainly by children who are inquisitive and drink apparently innocent-looking items, e.g. bleach, disinfectant and washing-up liquid. Always make sure items in the salon are clearly marked, i.e. surgical spirit, diluted antiseptic, nail varnishes and remover. If you are a home-visiting therapist and there are children in the house, ensure these items are out of their reach.

If poison has been taken, some of the following symptoms will occur:

1. pain in the stomach;
2. diarrhoea, retching or vomiting;
3. if the poison swallowed was corrosive, i.e. bleach, the lips and mouth will show white burns or blisters;
4. difficulty in breathing;
5. delirium and convulsions;
6. unconsciousness.

Anyone suspected of swallowing poison should be conveyed to hospital as quickly as possible. If the person is conscious, try to find out what has been swallowed. Look around to see if there is a bottle or container. Do not cause vomiting as it wastes time and could cause further harm. If you believe the person has swallowed a corrosive substance and is of course conscious, you can give about a pint of milk or alternatively dissolve a teaspoon of sodium bicarbonate in a pint of water to drink slowly. This will help to dilute the substance in the stomach. If the person becomes unconscious and still breathing, place him/her in the recovery position. If the breathing shows signs of failing, apply artificial respiration. At all times keep the person warm until medical help arrives or during transit to the hospital.

Stings

Bee stings have acid venom and wasp stings contain alkali venom. A bee sting can be seen and removed with sterilised tweezers or needle, but be careful not to squeeze the poison bag, otherwise it will just spread more poison into the skin. Once this has been done the whole area can be treated with an anti-histamine cream or apply a solution of 1 tsp of bicarbonate of soda in a tumbler of water to the area.

Wasp stings are usually hard to find, so apply vinegar, lemon juice or a weak solution of ammonia (10% ammonia and 90% water) to the area to neutralise the venom.

Mosquitoes can be a nuisance in some areas. Cold water, surgical spirit or cologne may help. It is advisable to keep some antihistamine cream in the first-aid box.

Strokes

A stroke is not always easily recognised. A client may complain of a headache or have symptoms resembling intoxication. The latter appears to be the case if there is difficulty in speaking and swallowing and there is considerable confusion and drowsiness. A stroke is obvious if there is paralysis down one side of the body. This is due to a rupture or blockage of a blood vessel in the brain, depriving the brain of blood supply.

If the person is conscious, lay him/her down with the head and shoulders, supported by a pillow. Turn the head to one side to allow any saliva to run from the mouth. Under no circumstances should drinks be given. Telephone the client's doctor or dial 999 for an ambulance. Loosen all clothing around the neck, chest and waist.

If the person becomes unconscious, move him/her into the recovery position (see pp. 330–332).

Chapter 17

Careers in beauty therapy

There are many venues open to the qualified beauty therapist and the following is a brief guide.

As an employee

Often this is the best way to start a career as it enables the student to gain confidence in giving treatments and the ability to handle the public. There is always the possibility of learning new techniques, using different types of products and equipment. Opportunities arise in salons, leisure centres, health spas, cruise ships and occasionally attendance in hospitals and nursing homes.

Most salons will require you to work at least one evening a week and usually all day Saturday as this is normally the busiest day. It is important to be flexible, probably working longer hours, due to clients arriving late for appointments or emergencies (i.e. when another therapist falls sick) and it may be necessary to cover for holidays. Working schedules will vary according to the bookings taken, and during slack periods the salon will require cleaning and ensuring that a fresh supply of dry towels etc. is available. Stock levels will need checking and the employer advised when these are becoming low, not when you have taken the last pot or bottle out of stock!

In leisure centres the emphasis is more on health and fitness rather than on the beauty aspect of your work. It is important to have a thorough knowledge of diet and nutrition as well as the effects of exercise.

Working in a health spa or farm usually means being part of a team but is often invaluable as it enables you to use all aspects of your beauty therapy training.

Most cruise ships or ocean liners have a salon on board combining hairdressing with beauty therapy. The work involved is rather limited to facials, manicures, pedicures and body massages. It is very appealing to the therapist, a chance to see other parts of the world and meet people of many nationalities. The rules on board the ship are very strict, usually confining staff to certain areas and your shared cabin is normally in the bowels of the ship, often without a port-hole – not for the claustrophobic therapist! The pay is not very good but gratuities are both a recognised and substantial source of income.

Attendance in a hospital or nursing home is usually on an *ad hoc* voluntary basis, giving treatments such as cosmetic camouflage, epilation or helping clients before or after cosmetic surgery.

To have rights as an employee you must work 16 hours per week or have worked 8 hours per week for 5 years, however, government legislation changes periodically and advice can always be obtained at a Citizens Advice Bureau (CAB).

The employee should receive a Contract of Employment which must be given within 13 weeks of employment and this should include:

- the hours of work, the wage per hour or salary per week/month;
- the duties and the responsibilities involved, i.e. job title;
- sickness pay;
- payment for overtime or hours off in lieu;
- holiday entitlement and the number of bank holidays given;
- the length of notice required to terminate employment.

There are various other particulars which you should expect to receive, i.e. an itemised pay slip. For a female employee, you are entitled to attend ante-natal care with pay and maternity pay with the option of returning to work after maternity leave, if you have been employed for a certain length of time (check with the CAB). You are not entitled to be unfairly dismissed and you should always be given a written statement for reasons of dismissal.

As a self-employed therapist

More and more beauty therapists have the urge to go into business for themselves and, as a travelling therapist, making visits to the clients' homes, it presents the opportunity to be self-employed without the overheads of owning a salon. Travelling by public transport will undoubtedly limit the type of treatments that can be given; therefore a reliable car or van is desirable for the carrying of equipment. There are distinct tax advantages in buying a van and no doubt your accountant will explain these to you. Many women appreciate this service, especially if they are house-bound or have a reluctance to discuss figure faults or undergo treatments in a salon.

Before embarking on this type of service the therapist should consult the local council's licensing office to check whether a licence is required for visiting services. Local authorities vary considerably but some will ask to see certificates or diplomas to ensure that you are qualified for this purpose.

As you are treating members of the public you must have public liability insurance and it is wise to shop around the various insurance companies or local insurance broker's office for the best quotation for the best cover. Other insurances you may consider are product liability or a replacement policy. The former will protect you if an accident occurs due to faulty equipment or by products used. The latter comes into effect if equipment or products are stolen or lost, where the insurance company will pay the *original* cost of the item.

As a self-employed person, your tax and National Insurance must be paid out of income. It is unlikely that you will need to be registered for VAT (Value Added Tax), but your accountant will advise you and also help you to set up your books, work out your tax problems and may even help with the pricing of your services.

There are many advantages as a travelling beauty therapist: there are no overheads, you can choose your own working hours, possibly to fit in with children or to dovetail with another job; you can also choose the area and the treatments you want to give. There are, of course, disadvantages, such as irregular and unsocial hours, petrol costs and car maintenance. There can be a communication problem which may lose you bookings, but this can be overcome by an answer-phone in the home or a car phone (some even have answer-phone facilities).

Undoubtedly there will be some initial expense and it is wise to talk to your bank manager but not before you have completed your market research and formed some sort of business plan. For the former the area chosen is vitally important, e.g. rural areas are very suitable for the mobile therapist, especially as clients need to travel into the towns where most salons are situated.

The equipment needed depends upon the services you intend to give, but initially this can be minimal, possibly starting with manicure and pedicure sets, depilatory waxing kit, facial products, a make-up box, cotton wool, tissues and towels. This can be extended to include a portable massage couch to enable you to give body treatments, i.e. massage, aromatherapy and the use of a faradic muscle toning machine and a vibratory massager.

There are manufacturers who specialise in practical portable beauty therapy equipment and these can be seen at conferences or exhibitions held regularly. Try to keep small items in a suitable box with a lid – many clients have inquisitive children who will enjoy putting their fingers in your precious creams or play with the make-up!

You also have the ideal opportunity to sell retail products but initially the range should be small until the business has grown and you can appreciate client requirements.

It is important to publicise your services; always have to hand a leaflet detailing these together with the prices charged, together with your name, address, telephone number and qualifications. Spread these leaflets around the area, request permission to pin them on notice boards in local factories, offices, social clubs, Women's Institutes, the Young Farmers Association or similar local groups (even some supermarkets or shops have notice boards).

Nearly every local newspaper has a women's page where you can insert a small advertisement or even write an article for the editor. There are also local radio stations looking for new material, where you could offer advice on many subjects to the public. All this requires an enthusiastic beauty therapist prepared to 'sell' her services and not sit at home waiting for the 'phone to ring! Working hard, maintaining professional standards and giving a good service will soon result in personal recommendations from clients which will enable your business to expand.

Another way to be self-employed is to take spare space in a hairdressing salon. You should establish at the outset your overheads, the cost of rent, whether it is paid weekly, monthly or quarterly; whether it includes electricity, or if there is a separate meter for the beauty salon. With the introduction of water meters, are you expected to make any contribution to the cost or pay anything towards the water rate or business rate levied? Does the salon owner expect any part of your profits?

As with any business agreement there are advantages and disadvantages. For the former there could be a ready-made clientèle and it may be possible to share the costs of advertising, or use the same receptionist for booking treatments as well as making hair appointments. The disadvantages could be keeping the same hours as the hairdressing salon; you could be situated at the back of the salon and you may have to take clients all through the hair salon first and the latter may also be noisy.

As an employer

For this purpose it is essential to learn the basic forms of business organisation which can be adopted and these include *sole trader, partnership*, and *various types of company*.

A sole trader   enters a business on his/her own account, obtaining the capital to start up the business, working with or without the aid of employees and as a reward receives the proceeds of the venture. There are very few formal procedures required for this type of business organisation but an accountant and liaison with the bank manager are necessary. However, it should be remembered that to make a profit, and this is important to expand or even cover overheads, you will need to work long hours, take few holidays, and realise that sickness could lead to difficulties and that you are personally liable to the full extent of your private funds for the debts of the business.

A partnership   can be formed with no legal formalities but it is wise to draw up a deed of partnership to include the names of the partners and the business; the amount of money each partner contributes; the ratio in which profits or losses are to be accepted; in which manner the accounts will be kept and the duration of the partnership. There is a Partnership Act 1980 which lays down certain rights and duties and your solicitor will advise you on these. Again you should be aware that all partners are liable for all debts and obligations incurred by the business.

Various types of company   include a public limited company (plc) or a private limited company. It is rather doubtful that you will be concerned with the former but you may be interested in the latter where the company formed must have at least one director and a company secretary who must be separate people, although the secretary may also be a director. Professional advice should be sought for the formation and registration of the company to include the Memorandum and Articles of Association and a certificate of trading must be obtained from the Register of Companies. The directors are only liable for the amount of money invested in the company by way of shares, providing that the business has been conducted in a proper manner.

In starting your own business you must consider the following.

1. Firstly and most importantly you must ask yourself if you are the sort of person who should be going into business. Are you, and possibly your family, prepared for the hard work, long hours and the strain that are involved in a start-up situation? Another question to ask yourself is: do you have sufficient commercial know-how?
2. Research the market to establish if there is any gap for your services. Obtain as many facts as possible – look at the competition and ask yourself if you are offering potential customers exactly what they want.
3. Pricing: get the price right. Will your clients pay a price that will still provide you with a sufficient profit margin? To start with, you may consider a pricing structure with room for discounts if needed.
4. You will need premises to operate from. Ensure that they are in the right location, affordable, in reasonably good condition and suitable for your business requirements.
5. Staff – if you need to employ people, choose with care. It is essential that you have the right people with the right skills.
6. Marketing – this is too often a neglected side of the business. You will need to persuade potential clients to favour your establishment. How are you going to do this? What support will you need from advertising, brochures, etc.?
7. Find out what grants may be available to you for capital expenditure, training, professional advice, etc. Sometimes, unsecured or 'soft' loans may be available.
8. Make arrangements to keep proper accounting records so that you can compare your actual trading position against your budgets. You will also need to register in good time for PAYE and VAT.
9. Prepare projections. Having considered all that it takes to start up and run your own business, convert it into detailed projections of both profit and cash flow. The projections will show if you will make enough money to sustain the business and reveal the amount of finance required. Be realistic and allow for contingencies, bearing in mind that costs are always easier to project than income.
10. If you need outside finance – for example, from a bank or third party – then you must prepare a business plan which should cover all the points previously mentioned. A well-conceived business plan is vital when you need to raise capital – whether from a bank or partner. The content and quality of presentation of the plan is critical in persuading an interested party that:

● the project is viable; and
● you are capable of running the business.

It is important for you to take out various insurances to cover your business activities, premises, equipment, etc., in case of fire, theft, water damage and a professional indemnity policy to cover you and your staff should a claim arise from a client.

This is a very cursory glance at starting up your own business but you are advised to read the many books written by eminent authors on business organisation, marketing and public relations to further your theoretical knowledge at least and to keep up-to-date with the various practices and the law, and to ensure that your business has every opportunity to succeed.

Index